Chang

Clinical Management of

Communication Problems

in Adults with

Traumatic Brain Injury

THE REHABILITATION INSTITUTE OF CHICAGO
PUBLICATION SERIES
Don A. Olson, Ph.D., Series Coordinator

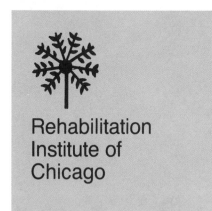

Rehabilitation
Institute of
Chicago

Clinical Management of Communication Problems in Adults with Traumatic Brain Injury

Anita S. Halper, MA, CCC-SP
Director, Department of Communicative Disorders
Rehabilitation Institute of Chicago
Assistant Professor
Assistant Professor, Clinical Physical Medicine and Rehabilitation
Northwestern University Medical School
Chicago, Illinois
Clinical Assistant Professor
Department of Communication Sciences and Disorders
Northwestern University
Evanston, Illinois

Leora R. Cherney, PhD, CCC-SP
Clinical Researcher
Department of Communicative Disorders
Rehabilitation Institute of Chicago
Assistant Professor
Clinical Physical Medicine and Rehabilitation
Northwestern University Medical School
Chicago, Illinois

Trudy K. Miller, MA, CCC-SP
Clinical Supervisor
Department of Communicative Disorders
Rehabilitation Institute of Chicago
Chicago, Illinois

AN ASPEN PUBLICATION®
Aspen Publishers, Inc.
Gaithersburg, Maryland
1991

Library of Congress Cataloging-in-Publication Data

Halper, Anita S.
Clinical management of communication problems in adults with traumatic
brain injury / Anita S. Halper, Leora R. Cherney, Trudy K. Miller.
p. cm. — (The Rehabilitation Institute of Chicago publication series)
Includes bibliographical references and index. ISBN: 0-8342-0279-4
1. Communicative disorders. 2. Brain damage—Patients—Rehabilitation.
I. Cherney, Leora Reiff. II. Miller, Trudy K. III. Title. IV. Series.
[DNLM: 1. Brain Injuries—complications. 2. Brain Injuries—rehabilita-
tion. 3. Communicative Disorders—etiology. 4. Communicative
Disorders—rehabilitation. WL 354 H195c]
RC423.H3238 1991
617.4'81044—dc20
DNLM/DLC
for Library of Congress
91-22270
CIP

The authors have made every effort to ensure the accuracy of the information
herein, particularly with regard to drug selection and dose. However, appropriate
information sources should be consulted, especially for new or unfamiliar drugs
or procedures. It is the responsibility of every practitioner to evaluate the
appropriateness of a particular opinion in the context of actual clinical situations
and with due consideration to new developments. Authors, editors, and the
publisher cannot be held responsible for any typographical or other errors found
in this book.

Editorial Services: Barbara Marsh

Library of Congress Catalog Card Number: 91-22270
ISBN: 0-8342-0279-4

Printed in the United States of America

1 2 3 4 5

Table of Contents

Contributors

James R. Andrews, PhD
Professor and Director of Clinical Services
Department of Communicative Disorders
Northern Illinois University
Dekalb, Illinois

Mary A. Andrews, MS
Instructor
Department of Communicative Disorders
Northern Illinois University
Dekalb, Illinois
Couple and Family Therapist
Kairos Family Center
Elgin, Illinois

Foreword

The problems of the traumatically brain injured have been with us for many, many years. However, only recently have the comprehensive needs of this population begun to be understood by individual, private and federal agencies. Further, the rehabilitation potential, the eventual outcomes and the total ramifications of this disability are yet to be well documented. As we gain more knowledge about this area, it becomes increasingly apparent that far too many individuals needing rehabilitation services, and in particular, speech and language services, are not finding them.

Medical advances have greatly improved the physical recovery of many individuals following traumatic brain injury, but the same level of improvement has not been achieved in the psychosocial, educational, vocational, and speech and language areas. Major challenges in this area center around lack of knowledge of head injuries, financial barriers, insufficient programs for injury prevention and treatment, and most importantly, limited access to appropriate rehabilitation re-

sources. Traumatic brain injured individuals and their families have tremendous challenges. In far too many rehabilitation situations, available resources staff and therapists have not been able to rise to those challenges.

This book is based on the premise that there is hope and change possible for the traumatically brain injured individual. Hope and change in the communicative disorders area can best occur when a program of comprehensive clinical management is developed and adhered to. The rehabilitation model presented in this book focuses on the individual and his family, since traumatic brain injury affects the lives of both in an equal fashion. Functional outcomes can only be achieved with a comprehensive, coordinated approach to the problem which builds cooperation between the rehabilitation team, the individual, his family, and the community to which the individual will return.

The authors of this book are experienced clinicians with years of experience working with the traumatically brain injured. This book describes a practical, functional, and proven approach to maximizing the potential of traumatically brain injured individuals.

These approaches are grounded on a scientific basis which has been proven by the experience and research of the authors. This text is a needed addition to the library of any Speech-Language-Cognitive Therapists working with this population.

Don A. Olson, PhD
Director
Education and Training Center
Rehabilitation Institute of Chicago
Associate Professor
Departments of Physical Medicine
    and Rehabilitation and Neurology
Northwestern University Medical
    School
Chicago, Illinois

Preface

Interest in the rehabilitation of persons with traumatic brain injury (TBI) has flourished over the past ten years. It is estimated that more than two million head injuries occur annually in the United States, with about 500,000 being admitted to the hospital.[1] Advances in medical technology have resulted in increasing numbers of survivors. Communication problems are a frequent sequelae of TBI. In fact, Sarno[2,3] found that all 125 TBI patients consecutively admitted to a rehabilitation hospital over a ten-year period displayed some degree of communication impairment. Speech-language pathologists in a variety of settings are faced with the management of the communication problems of such patients.

Clinical Management of Communication Problems in Adults with Traumatic Brain Injury grew out of a need to provide a comprehensive and structured approach to the development and implementation of treatment plans and to the documentation of progress. This book does not address specific management of aphasia, dysarthria, and dysphagia, but rather focuses on the cognitive-linguistic problems that are unique to the TBI population. A major focus has been to propose a framework on which subsequent evaluation and treatment guidelines can be based. An annotated compendium of selected evaluation tools and treatment/computer materials is provided as a reference source for the practicing clinician. These are intended as a guide and should be used only after careful analysis of the specific patient's strengths, weaknesses, premorbid levels of functioning, and needs. The role of the family or significant others as an integral part of the rehabilitation process is also discussed.

The book is divided into six chapters. In Chapter 1, Cherney discusses the neuropathology of traumatic brain injury and summarizes the literature as it relates to our framework for treatment. Cherney and Miller, in Chapter 2, discuss a method of classifying the cognitive, linguistic, motor speech production, and feeding problems in the traumatic brain injured population. A framework underlying clinical management is presented in Chapter 3 by Halper, Cherney, and Miller. In Chapter 4, Miller, Halper, and Cherney present guidelines for evaluating the cognitive-linguistic processes described in the previous chapter. In Chapter 5, Cherney, Halper, and Miller present goals, procedures, and measures for each of the processes described. In Chapter 6, Andrews and

Andrews present a paradigm for services which support family participation and specific techniques for involving the family on the rehabilitation team.

It is our hope that speech-language pathologists will find this book helpful in daily clinical practice and that it will be a welcome addition to their texts on traumatic brain injury.

REFERENCES

1. Goldstein M. Traumatic brain injury: a silent epidemic. *An Neurol.* 1990;27:327.
2. Sarno MT. The nature of verbal impairment after closed head injury. *J Nerv Men Dis.* 1980;168:685–692.
3. Sarno MT. Verbal impairment after closed head injury. *J Nerv Men Dis.* 1984;172:475–479.

Acknowledgments

The authors would like to thank Shelley I. Mogil for her contributions to Chapter 4, "Evaluation of Communication Problems in the Traumatic Brain Injured Adult." We are also grateful to the staff of the Department of Communicative Disorders at the Rehabilitation Institute of Chicago for their comments on Chapter 5, "Treatment of Communication Problems in the Traumatic Brain Injured Adult." A special note of thanks to Don Olson, PhD, Director of Education and Training, for his continued support of the publications in the Communicative Disorders Department.

Chapter 1

Cognitive-Linguistic Problems Associated with Traumatic Brain Injury: A Perspective

Leora R. Cherney

There is general agreement that communication disorders are an integral part of the multiplicity of deficits that result from traumatic brain injury (TBI) and that these deficits tend to persist over time. However, there are differences of opinion regarding the exact nature of the impairment. In order to understand the cognitive-linguistic sequelae of TBI, it is helpful to review the neuropathological mechanisms of cerebral trauma. Following this, the pertinent literature supporting the proposal that a cognitive basis underlies the communication deficits associated with TBI is discussed. Based on this viewpoint, Chapter 3 will propose a framework that has important implications for evaluation and treatment.

THE NEUROPATHOLOGY OF TRAUMATIC BRAIN INJURY

At the outset, it is important to differentiate between two types of brain damage—primary and secondary.[1,2] Primary brain damage occurs at the time of injury and is related to the mechanical forces present at the moment of impact. It is usually permanent, is seldom affected by treatment, and is the major factor that limits recovery. Primary damage results in two different types of lesions: contusions, which tend to be more discrete, and diffuse axonal injury, which tends to be more diffuse.

Secondary brain damage refers to the pathologic processes that occur in the brain as a result of the primary brain damage. Secondary damage may be intracranial, such as edema, hemorrhage, hematomas, infection, or hydrocephalus; or it may result from injuries to other parts of the body, such as respiratory failure from chest injuries. Regardless of the type of secondary problem, the ultimate mechanism responsible for damage to the brain is either hypoxia/ischemia or distortion and compression of the brain.[1] Anoxic damage occurs most commonly in the hippocampus, the basal ganglia, and the watershed areas of the cerebral cortex and the cerebellum.[3]

Secondary damage may occur several hours or even days or weeks after the primary injury. Unlike primary brain damage, secondary brain damage is potentially preventable or reversible with medical treatment. For instance, a hematoma can be surgically removed, or hydrocephalus can be treated with placement of a shunt to decrease intracranial pressure. Once the potential cause of secondary brain damage has been dealt with, some recovery of function can be anticipated.[1] Secondary problems should not be overlooked, since their effects may be additive to the direct effects of primary brain damage. However, when patients are treated optimally in the acute care setting, the effects of secondary brain damage are usually minimal.[4] Therefore, this section focuses on types of primary damage and the clinical implications for rehabilitation and does not further address the types of secondary damage.

Contusions

Contusions are bruises that occur over the surface of the brain. They initially look hemorrhagic and swollen, but later appear as small scars.[5] In an open or penetrating head injury, in which there is discontinuity of the meninges and often an associated skull fracture, contusions may occur at the site of impact.[6] However, in a closed or non-penetrating head injury, an important feature of cerebral contusions is that they occur in predictable locations, independent of the site or direction of the initial impact.[7,8] The areas involved are the undersurfaces of the frontal lobe and the anterior poles of the temporal lobe. Contusions are rarely seen in the occipital lobe. Additionally, contusions are typically bilateral and asymmetrical.[9,10]

The predictable location of contusions can be explained because of the peculiarities of the skull–brain interface.[11,12] Traumatic brain injury induces relative movement between the brain and the skull. As the incompressible brain moves, it makes contact with the inside of the rigid skull. The internal contour of the skull is irregular and jagged, particularly in the areas of the anterior and middle cranial fossa, where the crista galli of the ethmoid bone and the greater wing of the sphenoid bone are located. Therefore contusions typically occur in the frontal and temporal regions where the brain hits against these bony protuberances.

Research has shown that there is no correlation between the severity of contusions and loss of consciousness.[1,13] Depending on the location and extent of the contusions, the patient may demonstrate more localizing neurological signs such as hemiplegia and aphasia.

Diffuse Axonal Injury (DAI)

While cerebral contusions occur more commonly in falls and direct blows to the head, diffuse axonal injury is seen most commonly in high speed acceleration and subsequent deceleration injuries, such as motor vehicle accidents.[14] The head need not actually strike a surface for DAI to occur.[12] When a vehicle stops suddenly, the sudden deceleration sets up a force that causes the brain to continue to accelerate rotationally. This rotational acceleration causes movement between different components of the brain. Movement of one part of the brain relative to another results in stretching of the neuronal fibers that interconnect the different brain regions. If the fibers are stretched too far, they will tear.[11] These microscopic lesions can accumulate and become extensive, eventually leading to tissue loss and atrophy. DAI is widespread but most frequently occurs in the deep white matter and in the brain stem.[6,13]

The severity of DAI correlates with the severity of loss of consciousness[15] and post-traumatic amnesia,[16] both of which are important considerations for rehabilitation. The duration of loss of consciousness reflects varying degrees of DAI. In an attempt to quantify level of consciousness, the Glasgow Coma Rating Scale was developed.[17] This scale, which is described further in Chapter 4, evaluates the stimuli required to induce eye opening, the best motor response, and the best verbal response. Based on these criteria, coma is defined as absence of eye opening, inability to obey commands, and failure to utter recognizable words. Such patients would receive a score of eight or less from a possible maximum score of 15. When coma is deep and persistent, axonal damage is severe and widespread. At the other end of the continuum is concussion, a brief loss of consciousness followed by prompt recovery without any localizing neurological signs.[18] DAI may result in concussion when most fibers escape permanent structural damage; they may be stretched but not torn.[1]

Post-traumatic amnesia (PTA) is also associated with the degree of diffuse damage. PTA is the interval between the time of the injury and the return of continuous memory for ongoing events. A patient with PTA can be alert and functioning, but have persistent severe deficits in retaining new information and processing new memories.[16] It is obvious that such deficits can contribute to disorientation and affect the ability to learn compensatory strategies.

While contusions and diffuse axonal injury occur as a result of two different mechanisms, and their severities do not correlate,[11,15] there is usually some degree of co-occurrence. Contusions and diffuse axonal injury are often seen together, with one or the other type of injury predominating. Depending on the extent and severity of each, different types of problems in language, cognition, speech, or swallowing may be present. It is important for the speech-language pathologist to differentiate disorders typical of focal lesions from those general cognitive deficits that are characteristic of diffuse injury. One type of deficit may be masked by the other. The difficulties in pinpointing and diagnosing the communication problems associated with TBI are evident in many early studies on communication problems in TBI.

COGNITIVE-LINGUISTIC DEFICITS IN TRAUMATIC BRAIN INJURY

Is It an Aphasia?

Historically, the speech-language pathologist trained in the treatment of aphasia was the professional involved in the management of communication problems in TBI. As a result, communication was typically evaluated using tests specifically designed for the aphasic population. The term aphasia was used in its broadest sense to refer to a neurogenic communication breakdown with reductions in the language modalities of auditory comprehension, oral expression, reading comprehension, and written expression.

Many investigators noted, however, that there were qualitative differences between the language of aphasia and that of TBI. Groher[19] found that although patients displayed elements of both aphasia and confused language disturbance in the acute stages of recovery, the specific aphasic component quickly resolved. The patient was left with

what Halpern and his associates[20] termed "the language of confusion." Milton, Prutting and Binder[21] found that the discourse of head injured patients was characterized by difficulties with prosody and affect. Decreased range of topic selection, decreased topic maintenance, and reduced turn taking were noted. The patients also displayed problems with the quantity and conciseness of their discourse, tending to be redundant or overdetailed. Prigatano and colleagues[22] identified problems of talkativeness, tangential verbalizations, and unusual and bizarre phrases as three nonaphasic language disturbances characteristic of TBI. These affected the patient's ability to communicate effectively in both social and vocational settings.

Such descriptions prompted speech-language pathologists to question whether the communication problems in TBI were truly an aphasia. Holland[23] noted that language facility tends to be relatively unaffected in TBI; rather, the residual deficits tend to be those of communicative competence and a result of more pervasive memory and cognitive deficits. Consequently, she stated that "if the language problems seen in closed head injured patients don't look like aphasia, sound like aphasia, act like aphasia, feel, smell or taste like aphasia, then they aren't aphasia."[23(p345)] Since that time, there is a growing body of literature that supports the contention that while aphasia, in the classic definition of the word, exists in a small number of TBI patients,[24–29] the majority of them exhibit deficiencies that extend beyond this definition.

Cognitive-Linguistic Disorders

Hagen[30,31] contends that the language impairments after TBI should be diagnosed and treated as part of an underlying cognitive disorganization. Language processing is supported by the cognitive processes of attention, discrimination, maintenance of temporal ordering of groups of stimuli, memory, categorization and association of stimuli, and part-to-whole and whole-to-part integration/synthesis of stimuli. Language impairment is a symptom of dysfunction of these cognitive processes. Communication difficulties such as irrelevant, confabulatory, circumlocutory, and tangential responses that lack logical and sequential order result from deficits in these cognitive processes.

Similarly, Adamovich, Henderson, and Auerbach[4] have suggested that the diffuse brain lesions secondary to TBI can result in information processing difficulties, cognitive deficits, and neurophysiological disorders. All affect the ability to communicate effectively. Information processing difficulties interfere with individual's ability to perceive, discriminate, organize, recall, and solve problems using good judgment. Generalized cognitive deficits result in inability to deal with ideas and perceptions beyond a specific level of difficulty. Neurophysiological disorders are characterized by difficulties with attention and recall that can lead to disorientation, disorganization, confusion, and bizarreness or confabulation.

With the growing emphasis on cognitively based communication problems, the American Speech-Language-Hearing Association addressed the role of the speech-language pathologist in the treatment of cognitively impaired individuals. The 1987 report of the subcommittee on language and cognition[32] stated that the interrelationship between cognition and language serves as the basis for effective communication. Therefore, a cognitive impairment can result in communication breakdown. Cognitively based disorders of communication were referred to as cognitive-communicative impairments, and specific cognitive impairments which might affect language were listed. These included: impaired attention, perception, and/or memory; inflexibility, impulsivity, and/or disorganized thinking or acting; inefficient processing of information; difficulty processing abstract information; difficulty learning new information, rules, and procedures; inefficient retrieval of old or stored information; ineffective problem solving and judgment; inappropriate or unconventional social behavior; and impaired "executive" functions such as goal-setting, planning, self-initiating, and self-monitoring.

More recently, Kennedy and DeRuyter[33] have recommended the use of the term cognitive-language disorders to describe the deficits following TBI. First, this term more accurately reflects the cause of the impairment, which includes both cognitive and language processes. Second, inclusion of the term language is more precise because communication may refer to other disorders such as voice problems, dyspraxia, dysarthria, and impaired hearing.

MODELS OF COGNITION AND COMMUNICATION, AND IMPLICATIONS FOR TREATMENT

The differentiation between pure linguistic problems and cognitive-linguistic problems has important implications for evaluation and treatment. Intervention procedures developed for the aphasic population are not typically appropriate for the TBI population. There has been a need for a conceptual framework that will help organize the evaluation process and provide direction and structure to the selection of goals, objectives, and activities.

Functional Systems Models

The theoretical model of functional systems proposed by Luria[34,35] has had an important influence on the field of cognitive rehabilitation. According to this model, the brain is organized into three integrated functional units, which are essential to the execution of any cognitive task. The first unit is responsible for regulating the level of arousal and wakefulness and includes areas of the brain stem and other subcortical areas. The second functional unit receives, analyzes, and stores tactile, visual, auditory, and kinesthetic sensory information. For each type of sensory information, a primary sensory zone receives the information, a secondary zone organizes and further processes the information, and tertiary zones integrate the information from different areas. The second functional unit includes the surface of the brain, primarily the temporal and posterior areas. The third functional unit, which includes the frontal areas, programs actions and regulates behavior in accordance with the program. Luria has suggested that any observable behavior results from the basic processes working within each functional system. Any impairment of the basic processes disrupts the functional systems and results in changes in behavior. Accordingly, recovery of function can occur through a reorganization of functional systems. New learned connections are established through cognitive retraining exercises targeted at the source of the problems or the basic processes that have been disrupted.

Bracy[36] concurs that the impairments produced by brain injury are manifestations of impairments of basic cognitive processes. Treatment should be directed toward the basic processes that are impaired. He has expanded Luria's conceptualization of functional systems into four major areas. The first area is important in determining levels of arousal, alertness, and responsivity and is similar to the first functional unit of Luria. The second area is involved in sensation and the initial processing of sensory information. The third area includes those brain areas and functional processes involved with integration of sensory information, perception, conception, and memory. The final area is involved in response planning, general cognitive organization, execution of motor programs, and other executive functions. The model stresses the importance of the executive area which plays a role in every aspect of behavior.

There are other conceptions of the workings and interconnections of the cognitive mechanisms that address communicative functions, but with varying degrees of emphasis. Differences arise because definitions of cognition vary in scope, and there are disagreements about which processes lie in the province of cognitive rehabilitation. For instance, Szekeres and colleagues[37(p89)] have stated that "verbal behavior may be considered an aspect of cognitive functioning,[38,39] a function that is relatively autonomous of cognition[40] or a function that is related dynamically to cognition."[41,42]

Process-Specific Models

Sohlberg and Mateer[43] have developed a process-specific approach to cognitive rehabilitation in which treatment is oriented toward specific cognitive areas. Language is considered to be one of the cognitive process areas together with orientation, attention, memory, visual processing, executive function, reasoning, and problem solving. Each area is defined by a theoretically motivated model. It is assumed that these areas can be treated indi-

vidually and that they can be directly retrained and remediated. The essential rehabilitation strategy, then, is that a constellation of hierarchically related tasks, all of which target the same component of a particular cognitive process, are systematically and repeatedly administered. While independent models for each cognitive process are carefully developed, the investigators do not address the interaction of one process on another.

Interrelating Systems and Processes

In contrast, Hagen[30,31] stresses the relationship between communication and cognition in TBI. He has suggested that treatment of communication disorders be directed toward reorganization of the underlying cognitive processes rather than the abnormal language consequences of cognitive disorganization. He contends that as cognitive processes become more organized, commensurate improvement in phonological, semantic, syntactic, and verbal reasoning abilities can be anticipated.

Similarly, Szekeres, Ylvisaker, and associates[37,44] stress the dynamic interrelationships within the cognitive processes and systems. Based on information processing theories of cognition, they have proposed that there are three general aspects of cognition: component processes, component systems, and functional integrative performances. Component processes are those operations involved in taking in, interpreting, considering, and retrieving information and formulating output. They include attention, perception, memory/learning, organization, reasoning, and problem solving/judgment. Organized structures composed of basic and acquired processes and knowledge are called component systems and include working memory, long-term memory, the executive system, and the response system. Functional-integrative performance focuses on real life activities and refers to the complex interaction of the entire cognitive mechanism with the environment.

From this model, an eclectic view to rehabilitation is adopted. Rehabilitation of cognitive-linguistic disorders includes retraining specific component processes, teaching personal and environmental compensations, and training for functional daily activities. In addition, since the executive system is considered to have a crucial role in rehabilitation, metacognitive instruction is also important. Such instruction might include information about brain-behavior relationships, types of brain damage, and how each of the cognitive processes are affected. This helps increase the patient's awareness and understanding of the deficits. Without adequate executive control, intervention that targets specific cognitive or communicative deficits is unlikely to generalize to everyday functional activities.[45]

Similarly, Adamovich, Henderson, and Auerbach[4] have suggested that several different approaches to treatment are appropriate depending on the stage of recovery. These include stimulation or arousal and alerting followed by structured, goal-oriented programs or operative retraining. These programs use activities designed to facilitate attention, perception, discrimination, organization, memory, and higher level problem analysis and problem solving. Finally, home and community-oriented programs for generalization of independent functioning are recommended.

CONCLUSION

This chapter has reviewed the neuropathology of traumatic brain injury. Primary and secondary brain damage have been defined and the mechanisms resulting in contusions and diffuse axonal injury (the two types of primary brain damage) have been explained. The literature supporting the proposal that communication deficits in TBI result from cognitive impairments has been discussed, together with implications for treatment.

Although recent advances have promoted greater understanding of the cognitive-linguistic deficits in TBI, there is still a need to develop structured intervention programs and to evaluate the efficacy of the intervention strategies utilized. The selection of treatment activities and criteria for measuring patient progress should be based on a unifying conceptual framework of communication and its relationship to other cognitive processes. Chapter 3 proposes such a framework in which different cognitive and linguistic processes are interrelated and affect overall communicative and executive functions.

REFERENCES

1. Teasdale T, Mendelow D. Pathophysiology of head injuries. In: Brooks N, ed. *Closed Head Injury: Psychological, Social and Family Consequences.* New York, NY: Oxford University Press; 1984:4–36.

2. Pang D. Pathophysiologic correlates of neurobehavioral syndromes following closed head injury. In: Ylvisaker M, ed. *Head Injury Rehabilitation: Children and Adults.* Boston, Mass: College-Hill Press; 1985:4–70.

3. Brooke M, Uomoto JM, Mclean A, Fraser RT. Rehabilitation of persons with traumatic brain injury: a continuum of care. In: Beukelman DR, Yorkston KM, eds. *Communication Disorders Following Traumatic Brain Injury: Management of Cognitive, Language, and Motor Impairments.* Austin, TX: Pro-Ed; 1991:15–45.

4. Adamovich BB, Henderson JA, Auerbach S. *Cognitive Rehabilitation of Closed Head Injured Patients: A Dynamic Approach.* San Diego, Calif: College-Hill Press; 1985.

5. Adams JH, Graham DI, Gennarelli TA. Contemporary neuropathological considerations regarding brain damage in head injury. In: Becker DP, Povlishack JT, eds. *Central Nervous System Trauma Status Report—1985.* Washington, DC: National Institutes of Health—NINCDS; 1985.

6. Auerbach SH. Neuroanatomical correlates of attention and memory disorders in traumatic brain injury: an application of neurobehavioral subtypes. *J Head Trauma Rehabil.* 1986;1(3):1–12.

7. Adams JH, Scott G, Parker LS, Graham OI, Doyle D. The contusion index: A quantitative approach to cerebral contusions in head injury. *Neuropathol Appl Neurobiol.* 1980;6:319–324.

8. Ommaya AK, Grubb RL, Naumann RA. Coup and contrecoup injury: observation on the mechanics of visible brain injuries in the rhesus monkey. *J Neurosurg.* 1971;35:503–516.

9. Clifton GL, Grossman RG, Makala ME, et al. Neurological course and computerized tomography findings after severe closed head injury. *J Neurol Surg.* 1980;52:611–624.

10. Ommaya AK, Gennarelli TA. Cerebral concussion and traumatic unconsciousness: correlations of experimental and clinical observations on blunt head injuries. *Brain.* 1974;97:633–654.

11. Holbourne AHS. Mechanics of head injuries. *Lancet.* 1943;2:438–441.

12. Bigler ED. Neuropathology of acquired cerebral trauma. *J Learn Dis.* 1987;20:458–473.

13. Plum F, Posner JB. *The Diagnosis of Stupor and Coma.* 3rd ed. Philadelphia, Pa: FA Davis Co; 1980.

14. Adams JH, Graham DI, Murray LS, Scott G. Diffuse axonal injury due to non-missile injury in humans: an analysis of 45 cases. *Ann Neurol.* 1982;12:557–563.

15. Gennarelli TA, Thibault LE, Adams JH, et al. Diffuse axonal injury and traumatic coma in the primate. *Ann Neurol.* 1982;12:564–574.

16. Brooks DN. Disorders of memory. In: Rosenthal M, Griffith ER, Bond MR, Miller JD, eds. *Rehabilitation of the Head Injured Adult.* Philadelphia, Pa: FA Davis Co; 1983:185–196.

17. Teasdale G, Jennet B. Assessment of coma and impaired consciousness: a practical scale. *Lancet.* 1974;2:81–84.

18. Bakay L, Glasauer FE. *Head Injury.* Boston, Mass: Little Brown; 1980.

19. Groher M. Language and memory disorders following closed head trauma. *J Speech Hear Res.* 1977;20:212–223.

20. Halpern H, Darley FL, Brown JR. Differential language and neurologic characteristics in cerebral involvement. *J Speech Hear Dis.* 1973;38:162–173.

21. Milton SB, Prutting CA, Binder GM. Appraisal of communicative competence in head injured adults. In: Brookshire RH, ed. *Clinical Aphasiology Conference Proceedings.* Minneapolis, Minn: BRK Publishers; 1984:114–123.

22. Prigatano GP, Roueche JR, Fordyce DJ. Nonaphasic language disturbances after closed head injury. *Language Sciences.* 1985;1:217–229.

23. Holland AL. When is aphasia aphasia? The problem of closed head injury. In: Brookshire RH, ed. *Clinical Aphasiology Conference Proceedings.* Minneapolis, Minn: BRK Publishers; 1982:345–349.

24. Heilman K, Safron A, Geschwind N. Closed head trauma and aphasia. *J Neurol Neurosurg Psychiatry.* 1971; 34:265–269.

25. Thomsen, IV. Evaluation and outcome of aphasia in patients with severe closed head trauma. *J Neurol Neurosurg Psychiatry.* 1975;38:713–718.

26. Levin HS, Grossman RG, Kelly PJ. Aphasic disorder in patients with closed head injury. *J Neurol Neurosurg Psychiatry.* 1976;39:1062–1070.

27. Sarno MT. The nature of verbal impairment after closed head injury. *J Nerv Ment Dis.* 1980;168:685–692.

28. Sarno MT. Verbal impairment after closed head injury: report of a replication study. *J Nerv Ment Dis.* 1984;172:475–479.

29. Schwartz-Cowley R, Stepanik M. Communication disorders and treatment in the acute trauma center. *Top Lang Disord.* 1989;9:1–4.

30. Hagen C. Language disorders secondary to closed head injury: diagnosis and treatment. *Top Lang Disord.* 1981;1:73–87.

31. Hagen C. Language disorders in head trauma. In Holland A, ed. *Language Disorders in Adults.* San Diego, Calif: College-Hill Press; 1984:247–281.

32. American Speech-Language-Hearing Association, Subcommittee on Language and Cognition. The role of speech-language pathologists in the habilitation and rehabilitation of cognitively impaired individuals: a report of the subcommittee on language and cognition. *ASHA.* 1987;29:53–55.

33. Kennedy MRT, DeRuyter F. Cognitive and language bases for communication disorders. In: Beukelman DR, Yorkston KM, eds. *Communication Disorders Following Traumatic Brain Injury: Management of Cognitive, Language, and Motor Impairments.* Austin, Tex: Pro-Ed; 1991:123–190.

34. Luria AR. *The Working Brain: An Introduction to Neuropsychology.* New York, NY: Basic Books; 1973.

35. Luria AR. *Higher Cortical Functions in Man.* New York, NY: Basic Books; 1966.

36. Bracy OL. Cognitive rehabilitation: a process approach. *Cog Rehabil.* 1986;4:10–17.

37. Szekeres SF, Ylvisaker M, Cohen SB. A framework for cognitive rehabilitation therapy. In: Ylvisaker M, Gobble EMR, eds. *Community Re-entry for Head Injured Adults.* Boston, Mass: College-Hill Press; 1987:87–136.

38. Anderson J. *Language, Memory, and Thought.* Hillsdale, NJ: Lawrence Erlbaum Assoc; 1976.

39. Piaget J. Piaget's theory. In: Mussen PH, ed. *Carmichael's Manual of Child Psychology.* New York, NY: John Wiley and Sons; 1970;1.

40. Chomsky N. *Language and Thought.* New York, NY: Harcourt Brace Jovanovich; 1968.

41. Sapir E. *Language.* New York, NY: Harcourt Brace World; 1921.

42. Vygotsky LS; Hanfmann E, Vakan G, trans. *Thought and Language.* Cambridge, Mass: MIT Press; 1962.

43. Sohlberg MM, Mateer C. *Introduction to Cognitive Rehabilitation.* New York, NY: Guilford Press; 1989.

44. Szekeres SF, Ylvisaker M, Holland AL. Cognitive rehabilitation therapy: a framework for intervention. In Ylvisaker M, ed. *Head Injury Rehabilitation: Children and Adults.* Boston, Mass: College-Hill Press; 1985: 219–246.

45. Ylvisaker M, Szekeres S. Metacognitive and executive impairments in head-injured children and adults. *Top Lang Disord.* 1989;9:34–49.

Chapter 2

A Classification System for Cognitive, Linguistic, Speech, and Swallowing Disorders in the Traumatic Brain Injured Adult

Leora R. Cherney and Trudy K. Miller

Patients with traumatic brain injury are a heterogeneous group with multiple problems including cognitive, linguistic, speech, and swallowing disorders. It is essential that these deficits be accurately identified so that an appropriate treatment program can be developed. It is also important that the interdisciplinary team understands the exact nature of these deficits and their impact on the patient's total rehabilitation, including the physical, social, behavioral, and emotional components.

There is disagreement in the literature regarding the identification and description of the communication and swallowing deficits that result from traumatic brain injury.[1] Groher[1] has suggested that this disagreement is related to differences in patient selection and methods of assessing the communication deficits. Differences in terminology used to describe the communication problems also add to the confusion. As a result, there is no consensus as to the exact prevalence of these problems in the TBI population.

The first step in addressing these problems is to delineate a practical and replicable means of classifying the cognitive, linguistic, speech, and swallowing disorders that result from traumatic brain

injury. This chapter outlines the classification system used in the Department of Communicative Disorders at the Rehabilitation Institute of Chicago. Data are also presented to illustrate how the classification system has been used. Since the intent is not to discuss recovery over time, detailed information such as length of time since onset, age, and educational level has been omitted.

DESCRIPTIVE CATEGORIES

Cognitive and Linguistic Areas

Reduced Alertness/Arousal and Responsiveness Resulting in Severe Communication Deficits. This category refers to those patients who are unresponsive or demonstrate only occasional nonpurposeful and delayed responses to both verbal and nonverbal stimuli. Receptive and expressive language is absent and the patient cannot participate in any evaluation tasks. Speech and swallowing problems may or may not be present. Patients who emerge from this stage will usually present with one of the other cognitive and linguistic disorders discussed below.

Cognitive-Linguistic Deficits Associated with Traumatic Brain Injury

Communication deficits occur in TBI patients as a result of both cognitive and linguistic impairments and their interaction. The American Speech-Language-Hearing Association's Subcommittee on language and cognition[2] has identified the following cognitive impairments affecting language:

- impaired attention, perception, and/or memory
- inflexibility, impulsivity, and/or disorganized thinking or acting
- inefficient processing of information (rate, amount, and complexity)
- difficulty processing abstract information
- difficulty learning new information, rules, and procedures
- inefficient retrieval of old or stored information
- ineffective problem solving and judgment
- inappropriate or unconventional social behavior
- impaired executive functions: self-awareness of strengths and weaknesses, goal setting, planning, self-initiating, self-inhibiting, self-monitoring, and self-evaluating

The specific cognitive and linguistic impairments typical of patients with traumatic brain injury are discussed further in Chapter 3.

It is important not only to differentiate the type of cognitive-linguistic deficit associated with traumatic brain injury but also to evaluate the extent of the deficit. Severity ratings have been developed to assist the speech-language pathologist in assigning an overall level of functional communicative ability. The scales provide a means to document changes in patient performance. They also allow for the consistent assignment of ratings by different clinicians within one department or across different facilities. Table 2-1 summarizes the severity rating scale for patients with cognitive-linguistic deficits associated with traumatic brain injury.

Aphasia

Although the majority of TBI patients suffer diffuse cerebral damage resulting in more general cognitive-linguistic deficits, some may present with an aphasia resulting from more focal cerebral injury.[3–7] When patients present with language

Table 2-1 Severity Levels for Cognitive-Linguistic Deficits Associated with Traumatic Brain Injury and Right Hemisphere Dysfunction

Level	Description
1–Severe	Severe deficits in behavior and cognition prevent functional communication.
2–Moderately Severe	Functional communication is inconsistent.
3–Moderate	Communication is functional in simple, familiar contexts; however, behavior and cognitive deficits interfere with accuracy and appropriateness.
4–Mild to Moderate	Communication is generally accurate and appropriate in most everyday contexts; obvious errors are present in complex contexts.
5–Mild	Communication is accurate and appropriate in most situations; specific impairments become apparent in distracting settings or through structured assessment.
6–Minimal	Communicates in a full range of contexts but patient may note subtle deficits in integrative skills.

Source: Department of Communicative Disorders, Rehabilitation Institute of Chicago. Reprinted with permission.

problems that are characteristic of an aphasia, these problems are categorized according to the system established by Goodglass and Kaplan.[8] According to this classification, the eight distinct types of aphasia are: global aphasia, Broca's aphasia, Wernicke's aphasia, anomic aphasia, conduction aphasia, transcortical sensory aphasia, transcortical motor aphasia, and mixed nonfluent aphasia. These syndromes, with their unique cluster of symptoms, serve as "anchor points" for differential diagnosis so that not all patients with aphasia will fit cleanly into a specific category.[8] Therefore, if possible, the aphasia is classified according to the syndrome it most resembles. A description of the similarities to and differences from the assigned syndrome is also included. In addition to aphasia type, a severity rating scale (Table 2-2) for functional communication in aphasic patients is used.

Since patients with traumatic brain injury may present with both diffuse and focal brain damage, an aphasia may occur together with cognitive-linguistic deficits. In some cases, the aphasia may be so severe that these cognitive-linguistic deficits are not discernible or their extent cannot be determined. In other cases, the cognitive-linguistic def-

icits may constitute the primary disorder, but aphasic-like errors such as word retrieval deficits and verbal and literal paraphasias may also occur. These patients, therefore, are classified as having cognitive-linguistic deficits associated with traumatic brain injury as well as an aphasic component.

Communication Deficits Associated with Right Hemisphere Dysfunction

A small number of traumatic brain injured patients may sustain primarily unilateral right hemisphere damage. Communication deficits associated with right hemisphere dysfunction are characterized by deficits in the areas of attention, orientation, perception, pragmatics, memory, and integration.[9] It is often difficult to differentiate this group of patients from those with the more general cognitive-linguistic deficits associated with traumatic brain injury because the effects on functional communication are similar. However, left-sided neglect and the severity of the visual-perceptual and pragmatic problems are hallmarks of communication deficits associated with right hemisphere dysfunction.[10] The severity rating

Table 2-2 Aphasia Severity Levels

Level	Description
1–Severe	No usable speech or auditory comprehension.
2–Moderately Severe	All communication is through fragmentary expression; great need for inference, questioning, and guessing by the listener. The range of information that can be exchanged is limited, and the listener carries the burden of communication.
3–Moderate	Conversation about familiar subjects is possible with help from the listener. There are frequent failures to convey the idea, but patient shares the burden of communication with the examiner.
4–Mild to Moderate	The patient can discuss almost all everyday problems with little or no assistance. Reduction of speech and/or comprehension, however, makes conversation about certain material difficult or impossible.
5–Mild	Some obvious loss of fluency in speech or facility of comprehension, without significant limitation on ideas expressed or form of expression.
6–Minimal	Minimal discernible speech handicap; patient may have subjective difficulties that are not apparent to the listener.

Source: Reprinted from *The Assessment of Aphasia and Related Disorders*, ed 2 (p 28) by H Goodglass and E Kaplan with permission of Lea & Febiger, © 1983.

scale for functional communication is the same as that used for patients with cognitive-linguistic impairments and is presented in Table 2-1.

Speech Production

Dysarthria, a reduction in speech intelligibility and/or speech naturalness subsequent to neurological damage, is a frequent consequence of traumatic brain injury. The classification system used for the differential diagnosis of dysarthria has been adapted from that of Darley, Aronson, and Brown[11] and includes flaccid, spastic, ataxic, hypokinetic, hyperkinetic, and mixed spastic-flaccid dysarthrias. Two additional categories, undifferentiated dysarthria Group 1 and Group 2, have been included for those patients who cannot be assigned one of the above labels because of difficulty in testing or in interpreting the evaluation results. The diagnosis of dysarthria is made on the basis of both motor and acoustic characteristics. However, some TBI patients have obvious oral motor impairments but limited or absent phonation which prevent the evaluation of acoustic characteristics (undifferentiated group 1). At the other end of the continuum, some patients may present with acoustic deviations in the absence of confirmatory oral motor deviations; the acoustic deviations may be so mild that they cannot be assigned to a specific dysarthria type (undifferentiated group 2). Table 2-3 provides the overall severity rating scale for dysarthria based on the intelligibility of functional speech.

There is a group of patients who are usually intelligible but present with acoustic deviations at the laryngeal level only. These patients are categorized as having a dysphonia.

Dysphagia

Traumatic brain injured patients frequently have difficulty with oral nutritional intake.[12] Problems may be a result of anatomical and physiological involvement of the oropharyngeal mech-

---

Table 2-3 Speech Production Severity Levels

Level	Description
1–Severe	Unintelligible functional speech; inability to modify speech due to severe muscle impairment.
2–Moderately Severe	Functional speech is usually unintelligible but improves with repetition, decreased rate, exaggerated articulatory movements or other compensatory techniques.
3–Moderate	Spontaneous production of phrases and short sentences is usually intelligible. Intelligibility decreases as length of output increases.
4–Mild to Moderate	Functional speech is usually intelligible (at least 75%) but repetition may be required. Significant deviations in phonation (dysphonia/aphonia) may be present.
5–Mild	Functional speech is typically intelligible (90–100%) but speech does not sound normal due to mild deviations in respiration, phonation, articulation, resonance, and prosody.
6–Minimal	Functional speech is consistently intelligible although subjective difficulties may be experienced (e.g., perceived reduction in intelligibility due to fatigue, perceived change in speech from premorbid status).

Source: Rehabilitation Institute of Chicago, Functional Assessment Scale (RIC-FAS II). Chicago, Ill: Rehabilitation Institute of Chicago; 1989. Reprinted with permission.

anism and/or cognitive, linguistic, and behavioral deficits that interfere with the eating/feeding situation.[12] Table 2-4 shows the functional severity rating scale for oral intake. In assigning these ratings, the anatomic/physiologic information obtained from the videofluoroscopic examination are considered together with cognitive, linguistic, and behavioral factors.

PREVALENCE DATA

The purpose of this section is to illustrate the use of the classification system. The cognitive, linguistic, speech, and swallowing diagnoses on patients admitted with a medical diagnosis of traumatic brain injury over a two and one-half year period are presented. Data were compiled on a total of 360 patients who met the following criteria:

- 18 years of age or older
- no known history of any disorder affecting communication prior to the traumatic brain injury
- a minimum length of stay of two weeks to ensure a complete evaluation

Table 2-4 Functional Severity Levels for Oral Intake

Level	Description
1–Severe	All nourishment via alternate feeding method Nothing by mouth Trial oral intake by speech-language pathologist
2–Moderately Severe	Alternate feeding method as primary source of nourishment Limited, inconsistent success with oral intake Patient requires constant supervision Some team involvement but only speech-language pathologist introduces new items or techniques
3–Moderate	Alternate feeding may be withdrawn on a trial basis Fairly reliable oral feeding with prescribed diet of specific items Patient requires close supervision Nursing staff most involved, following instructions of speech-language pathologist Speech-language pathologist working on addition of new items to diet
4–Mild to Moderate	Fairly reliable oral feeding with defined level of food consistency Patient may have difficulty with clear liquids or solids Patient requires supervision, for which nursing staff take primary responsibility
5–Mild	Patient receives regular diet with some food restrictions Patient may require some special techniques or procedures to achieve successful oral intake Patient does not require close supervision
6–Minimal	Patient receives a regular diet with no restrictions No supervision required Occasional episodes of coughing with liquids or solids
7–Normal	Independent oral intake of all consistencies of food Safe and efficient swallowing competency

Source: Reprinted from *Clinical Evaluation of Dysphagia* (pp 41–42) by LR Cherney, CA Cantieri and JJ Pannell, Aspen Publishers, Inc, © 1986.

Upon admission, every patient was evaluated by a speech-language pathologist assigned to the TBI program. A standard battery of tests was used depending on the level of the patient. Test selection was made in accordance with the procedures described in Chapter 4. When testing was completed, diagnoses were assigned for the cognitive and linguistic areas, speech production, and dysphagia. Severity ratings were also assigned. To ensure consistency of assigned ratings, all ratings were reviewed by the clinical supervisor.

Inter-rater reliability has been established on the overall severity rating scales for speech and dysphagia. In addition, reliability of severity ratings for each language modality (e.g., auditory comprehension, oral expression, reading comprehension, written expression) has been established. The overall severity ratings for the cognitive and linguistic areas are derived from these individual modality ratings. Inter-rater reliability was accomplished as part of an institute-wide project to determine the reliability of the *Rehabilitation Institute of Chicago (RIC) Functional Assessment Scale*.[13] The primary speech-language pathologist conducted the initial evaluation which was observed by the clinical supervisor. The severity levels were then independently assigned by the clinician and the supervisor. Ratings were completed on a total of 30 adult patients. Better than 97 percent agreement between raters was achieved for all categories except speech production where 93 percent agreement was achieved.

Cognitive and Linguistic Areas

Figure 2-1 displays the distribution of patients in each of the four diagnostic categories. Forty patients (11 percent) showed reduced alertness/arousal and responsiveness resulting in severe communication deficits. However, the majority of the patients (81 percent) presented with cognitive-linguistic deficits associated with traumatic brain injury. Included in this group of patients were nine patients who also showed an accompanying aphasic component. Figure 2-2 displays how the patients with cognitive-linguistic deficits associated with traumatic brain injury were grouped by severity level. It can be seen that patients tended to

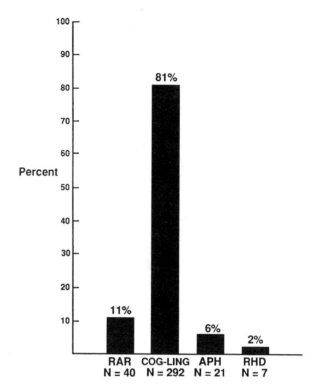

Figure 2-1 Prevalence of Cognitive and Linguistic Problems in TBI Patients (N = 360)

cluster at the severe end and middle of the continuum. At the upper end of the severity range, the number of patients decreased as severity decreased. This trend is typical of an acute rehabilitation facility which admits TBI patients in the early stages of recovery.

There is disagreement about the incidence of communication problems in TBI resulting from

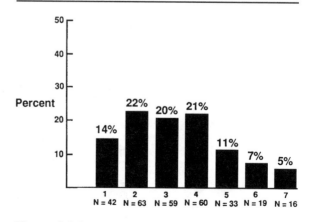

Figure 2-2 Severity of Cognitive-Linguistic Deficits Associated with TBI (N = 292)

unilateral brain damage. Only 8 percent of patients presented with communication problems indicative of focal cerebral damage. Two percent showed right hemisphere problems which, to our knowledge, have not been differentiated previously in patients with TBI. Classic aphasia resulting from focal left hemisphere problems was present in 6 percent of the patients. This number contrasts sharply with the 32 percent and 27.5 percent reported by Sarno[3,4] and the 24 percent reported by Thomsen.[14] These discrepancies may be a result of true differences in the patient sample or may reflect differences in the criteria used for classifying aphasia and the type of testing procedures utilized. The findings are more consistent with the 2 percent reported by Heilman and associates[6] and the 2.4 percent incidence of classical aphasia reported by Schwartz-Cowley and Stepanik.[15]

In an attempt to investigate the type of aphasia that occurs in traumatic brain injury, the 21 patients with aphasia were differentiated according to the type and severity of their aphasia (see Figures 2-3 and 2-4). These data demonstrate that traumatic brain injured patients present with many different types of aphasia. A greater proportion of the patients (62 percent) displayed a fluent aphasia which was primarily anomic or Wernicke's. This finding is consistent with previous reports. Heilmann and his colleagues[6] found that 9 of the 13 patients demonstrated anomic aphasia while Sarno[3,4] reported Wernicke's aphasia in the majority of TBI patients with aphasia. It is of interest to note that in the RIC data, the aphasia tended to be

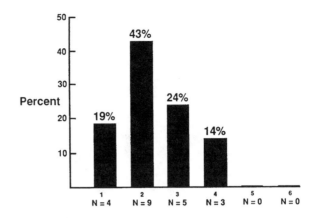

Figure 2-4 Severity of Aphasia (N = 21)

in the more severe range; no patients demonstrated mild to minimal aphasia.

Speech Production

The prevalence of dysarthria in traumatic brain injury is not well documented with estimates varying from 8 percent to 100 percent.[3,4,16–19] This broad range may be partly because of differences in the types of measures used, differences in the time at which the measures were taken,[19] and difficulties in conducting dysarthria evaluations. The RIC data were based upon the dysarthria assessments and subsequent intelligibility ratings that were assigned to only 297 of the 360 patients with traumatic brain injury. The presence of a dysarthria could not be determined in 63 patients because reduced alertness/arousal and responsiveness prevented sufficient assessment. Clinically, we have found that many of these patients exhibited a dysarthria when their level of responsiveness increased enough to permit a dysarthria evaluation. Of the remaining 297 patients, 56 (19 percent) displayed a dysarthria. An additional eight patients presented with voice disorders only and were diagnosed as having a dysphonia.

Figure 2-5 shows the distribution by dysarthria type. All types of dysarthria except hyperkinetic dysarthria were present. Of those patients in which a definitive diagnosis could be assigned, the most common types were flaccid (14 percent), spastic-flaccid (12.5 percent), and ataxic (11 percent). These findings are consistent with those of

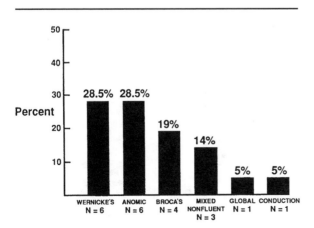

Figure 2-3 Types of Aphasia (N = 21)

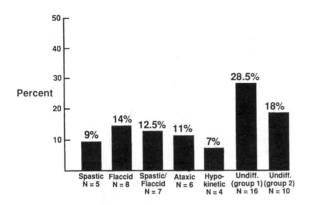

Figure 2-5 Types of Dysarthria (N = 56)

Groher[16] and Malkmus as reported by Groher.[1] Both investigators found the dysarthrias to be primarily flaccid, spastic, ataxic, or combinations of these three types of dysarthria. The large number of patients with undifferentiated dysarthria highlights the difficulty in assigning a dysarthria diagnosis. In 28.5 percent of the patients, there were obvious oral motor impairments but limited or absent phonation; 18 percent of the patients presented with acoustic deviations in the absence of confirmatory oral motor deviations.

Distribution of dysarthria by severity level is shown in Figure 2-6. All severity levels of dysarthria were present with large numbers clustering at the severe (30 percent) and mild/minimal (34 percent) ends of the continuum. Yorkston and colleagues[19] reported on severity levels of dysarthria in TBI patients in different clinical settings. They found that of 40 patients in an acute medical setting, 25 percent displayed non-

functional speech (intelligibility less than 20 percent) while 12.5 percent displayed moderate or mild dysarthria. In acute rehabilitation, 20 percent of 49 patients had nonfunctional speech while 45 percent had a moderate or mild dysarthria. In an outpatient rehabilitation setting, 10 percent of 62 patients had nonfunctional speech while 13 percent had a moderate or mild dysarthria.

Dysphagia

All 360 patients were assessed for dysphagia with 35 percent (127) displaying oral intake problems. This number is close to previous incidence findings of 27 percent to 30 percent of adult TBI patients having a dysphagia.[20-23] In contrast, Yorkston and associates reported a 77.5 percent incidence of swallowing problems in TBI patients in acute medicine, approximately 67 percent in acute rehabilitation, and 13 percent in outpatient rehabilitation.[19]

Figure 2-7 illustrates the distribution of the 127 patients according to functional severity levels for oral intake. The majority of these patients (66 per-

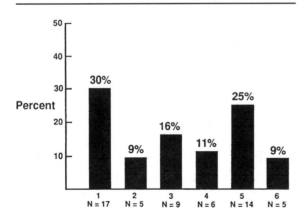

Figure 2-6 Severity of Dysarthria (N = 56)

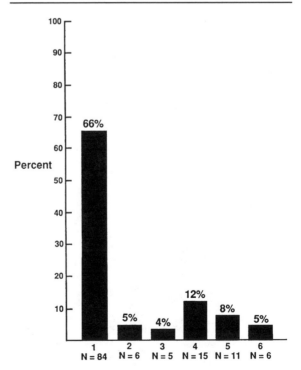

Figure 2-7 Severity of Dysphagia (N = 127)

cent) presented with severe dysphagia. This contrasts with the report of Lazarus and Logemann[22] in which 39.22 percent of the dysphagic TBI patients were rated as severe, 33.33 percent as moderate, and 27.45 percent as mildly dysphagic. Their study was based on only physiological severity levels defined by videofluoroscopy, without regard for cognitive, linguistic, and behavioral characteristics. It is important to consider these factors because in the TBI patient, oral intake skills and cognitive-linguistic skills are interdependent.[21]

Program Development

The data discussed reflect the patient population at RIC, an urban, acute rehabilitation center. Based on these data a comprehensive speech-language pathology program focusing on every aspect of the patients' care has been developed. Periodic review of these data has allowed for continuous revision of the speech-language pathology program in light of current trends in the hospital population. These data have been helpful in such areas as determining staffing requirements (e.g., increasing staff for feeding programs), budgetary needs (e.g., purchasing computers and appropriate software), and program development (e.g., introducing new group treatment formats).

CONCLUSION

This chapter has presented a practical means of classifying the cognitive, linguistic, speech, and swallowing disorders that result from traumatic brain injury. Data that represent the traumatic brain injured population in an urban rehabilitation center have been presented. There is a need for further studies that investigate the prevalence of cognitive, linguistic, speech, and swallowing problems in the TBI population across all settings. These studies should utilize consistent and replicable procedures for patient selection, identification and description of deficits, and the assignment of severity ratings. Such studies would identify more precisely the needs of patients at all stages of recovery and help with appropriate program and staff development.

REFERENCES

1. Groher ME. Communication disorders in adults. In: Rosenthal M, Griffith ER, Bond MR, Miller JD, eds. *Rehabilitation of the Adult and Child with Traumatic Brain Injury*. Philadelphia, Pa: FA Davis Co; 1990:148–162.

2. American Speech-Language-Hearing Association, Subcommittee on Language and Cognition. The role of speech-language pathologists in the habilitation and rehabilitation of cognitively impaired individuals: a report of the subcommittee on language and cognition. *ASHA*. 1987;29:53–55.

3. Sarno MT. The nature of verbal impairment after closed head injury. *J Nerv Ment Dis*. 1980;168:685–692.

4. Sarno MT. Verbal impairment after closed head injury: report of a replication study. *J Nerv Ment Dis*. 1984;172:475–479.

5. Thomsen IV. Evaluation and outcome of traumatic aphasia in patients with severe verified focal lesions. *Folia Phoniatri*. 1976;28:362–377.

6. Heilman K, Safron A, Geschwind N. Closed head trauma and aphasia. *J Neurol Neurosurg Psychiatry*. 1971;34:265–269

7. Levin HS, Grossman RG, Kelly PJ. Aphasic disorder in patients with closed head injury. *J Neurol Neurosurg Psychiatry*. 1976;39:1062–1070.

8. Goodglass H, Kaplan E. *The Assessment of Aphasia and Related Disorders*. Philadelphia, Pa: Lea and Febiger; 1983.

9. Burns MS, Halper AS, Mogil SI. Diagnosis of communication problems in right hemisphere damage. In: Burns MS, Halper AS, Mogil SI. *Clinical Management of Right Hemisphere Dysfunction*. Gaithersburg, Md: Aspen Publishers Inc; 1985:29–38.

10. Burns MS. Language without communication: the pragmatics of right hemisphere damage. In: Burns MS, Halper AS, Mogil SI. *Clinical Management of Right Hemisphere Dysfunction*. Gaithersburg, Md: Aspen Publishers Inc; 1985:17–28.

11. Darley FL, Aronson AE, Brown JR. *Motor Speech Disorders*. Philadelphia, Pa: WB Saunders; 1975.

12. Logemann JA. Preface. *J Head Trauma Rehabil*. 1989; 4:viii.

13. *Rehabilitation Institute of Chicago, Functional Assessment Scale (RIC-FAS II)*. Chicago, Ill: Rehabilitation Institute of Chicago; 1989.

14. Thomsen IV. Evaluation and outcome of aphasia in patients with severe closed head trauma. *J Neurol Neurosurg Psychiatry.* 1975;38:713–718.

15. Schwartz-Cowley R, Stepanik M. Communication disorders and treatment in the acute trauma center. *Top Lang Disord.* 1989;9:1–4.

16. Groher M. Language and memory disorders following closed head trauma. *J Speech Hear Res.* 1977;20:212–223.

17. Dresser AC, Meirowsky AM, Weiss GH, et al. Gainful employment following head injury: prognostic factors. *Arch Neurol.* 1973;29:111–116.

18. Rusk H, Block J, Lowman E. Rehabilitation of the brain injured patient: a report of 157 cases with long term follow-up of 118. In: Walker E, Caveness W, Critchley M, eds. *The Late Effects of Head Injury.* Springfield, Ill: Charles C Thomas; 1969:327–332.

19. Yorkston KM, Honsinger MJ, Mitsuda PM, Hammen V. The relationship between speech and swallowing disorders in head-injured patients. *J Head Trauma Rehabil.* 1989;4:1–16.

20. Winstein CJ. Neurogenic dysphagia: frequency, progression and outcome in adults following head injury. *Phys Ther.* 1983;12:1992–1997.

21. Cherney LR, Halper AS. Recovery of oral nutrition after head injury in adults. *J Head Trauma Rehabil.* 1989; 4:42–50.

22. Lazarus C, Logemann JA. Swallowing disorders in closed head trauma patients. *Arch Phys Med Rehabil.* 1987; 68:79–84.

23. Field LH, Weiss CJ: Dysphagia with head injury. *Brain Injury.* 1989;3:19–26.

Chapter 3

A Framework for Clinical Management

Anita S. Halper, Leora R. Cherney, and Trudy K. Miller

This chapter presents a conceptual framework for the clinical management of the cognitive-linguistic problems of adults with traumatic brain injury. This framework has been developed from clinical experience and the current neuropsychological and speech-language pathology literature discussed in Chapter 1.

Figure 3-1 is a schematic representation of the interrelationships among the different cognitive and linguistic processes. These processes include sensory reception, attention, perception, orientation, organization, reasoning, problem solving/judgment, semantics/pragmatics, and memory. The premise of the framework is that these processes underlie the performance of any task or functional behavior and must be considered in the selection of evaluation and treatment activities. Furthermore, rather than training the task or functional behavior, treatment should be directed toward improving the underlying processes that are impaired.[1–5] It is difficult to empirically evaluate the validity of this premise. However, the authors' collective clinical experience with hundreds of patients with traumatic brain injury indicates that this premise is clinically useful, practical, and effective. In the following section, each cognitive and linguistic process is defined and described.

Then, the interrelationships among the processes are discussed.

COGNITIVE AND LINGUISTIC PROCESSES

Attention

Attention is a complex process that affects all levels of cognitive processing. Alertness/arousal can be defined as the degree of wakefulness and level of responsiveness to stimulation. According to Mesulam,[6] there are two major components of attention: a basic matrix or state function and the more active vector or channel function. The matrix or state function determines the level of alertness/arousal, focusing capacity, and level of vigilance. It is associated with neuronal activity in the reticular formation.[6,7] The vector function is associated with more cortical activity and represents the active channeling of attentional processes toward a specific target. There is an interrelationship between these two components; in different tasks, one component may predominate over the other.

Sohlberg and Mateer[8] further delineate five levels of attention. These include focused and sus-

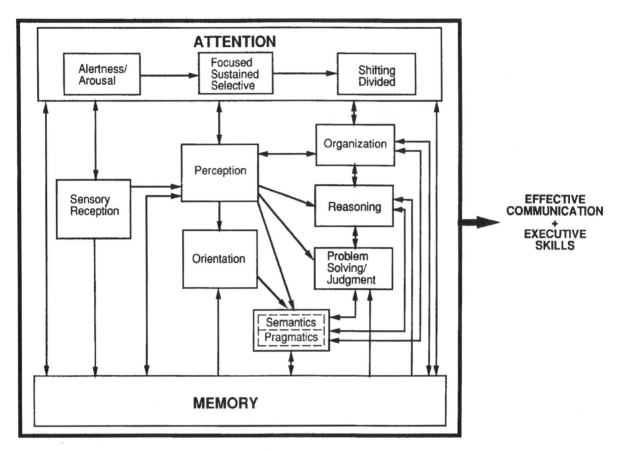

Figure 3-1 Cognitive and Linguistic Processes Affecting Communication and Executive Functions: A Clinical Framework

tained attention, which are mainly matrix functions, and selective, alternating, and divided attention, which are mainly vector functions. Focused attention is the ability to direct attention to specific sensory stimuli. Sustained attention involves actively maintaining attention to stimuli over a period of time. The ability to focus attention on target stimuli while ignoring irrelevant stimuli is selective attention. Alternating or shifting attention refers to the ability to move from one task to another task that requires different mental processes. Divided attention is the ability to simultaneously focus and sustain attention on more than one task. A basic level of alertness/arousal must be achieved before directing treatment activities toward improving focused and sustained attention. It is also assumed that the skills of focused, sustained, and selective attention must be present before one can shift and divide attention.

Sensory Reception and Perception

A process that is closely associated with alertness/arousal is sensory reception, the reception of tactile, visual, auditory, gustatory, olfactory, proprioceptive, and kinesthetic information.[9] Lezak[9] further states that sensory reception is a passive process that is responsible for activating the perceptual process. In contrast, perception is an active process that structures the environment by integrating sensory stimuli into meaningful units.[9] Perception includes such functions as identifying and discriminating salient features and detecting relationships and patterns.[10] The temporal and posterior cortical areas are primarily involved in the reception and perception of tactile, visual, auditory, and kinesthetic sensory stimuli.[7] Olfactory and gustatory information is processed in subcortical areas of the brain.[11]

Orientation

Orientation is the awareness of self in relation to person, place, situation, and time. Orientation to person is knowing oneself as well as others. Place (or geographic) orientation[12] includes being aware of where one is in the environment, finding one's way in familiar and new environments, and identifying places on maps or floor plans. Orientation to situation is the awareness of the present situation and the circumstances leading up to it. Orientation to time includes both telling time and monitoring the passage of time.

Higher Level Cognitive Processes

Organization, reasoning, and problem solving/judgment are so closely linked that it is difficult to separate them.[1] For effective functioning, each process relies to some extent on the other two processes. Organization is the ability to analyze and synthesize information, determine likenesses and differences, and sort, categorize, sequence, and prioritize information.

Reasoning is the ability to think abstractly and draw inferences and conclusions based on known or supposed information. Individuals reason in several ways. Inductive reasoning involves drawing conclusions from partial or indirect information. Deductive reasoning involves logically determining specific facts from a general premise or principle. In deductive reasoning, the analysis progresses from the whole situation to specific parts or features, while inductive reasoning requires an analysis of parts or details to formulate an overall concept.[1] A form of inductive reasoning is analogic reasoning which involves determining the relationship between similar situations and generalizing it to a new situation.

Reasoning has also been differentiated into convergent and divergent thinking. Convergent thinking is the analysis of information around a main idea or central topic.[1] Inductive and deductive reasoning are both types of convergent thinking.[13] Divergent thinking relates to flexibility of thought and is the creative generation of alternate ideas or interpretations.[13]

Problem solving requires both convergent and divergent thinking. It involves the following steps: recognizing and analyzing a problem; developing alternate solutions for solving the problem; evaluating the solutions; selecting the most appropriate solution; implementing the solution; and evaluating its effectiveness.[13,14] Judgment involves forming an opinion or estimate and predicting the consequences of an action based on known information.[13]

Memory

The three operations of memory are encoding, storage, and retrieval of information.[15] Encoding is the mechanism by which the representation of an event is acquired; storage is the retention of this representation over time. During retrieval, information is shifted from storage to a level of awareness. These three operations are necessary for learning new information.

Despite differences in terminology, there is a general consensus that memory can be divided into the three major components of sensory, short-term and long-term memory.[16] Sensory memory refers to the initial processing or encoding of information following registration by the sensory organs. If the sensory information is not transferred to short-term memory, it decays rapidly. Sensory memory is modality specific and has been referred to as iconic memory for visual stimuli and echoic memory for auditory stimuli.[15]

Short-term memory is the temporary storage system that holds information for a few seconds or minutes for either retrieval or transfer to the more permanent long-term memory store. Short-term memory has also been called primary memory,[17] immediate memory,[9] and working memory.[18] Working memory is a relatively new concept. Rather than a unitary system, it is conceived of as a collection of work areas where information is temporarily processed simultaneously.[18] Each cognitive processing system has its own working memory capacity[19] which is integrated by a central executive system.[18]

Long-term memory permanently stores knowledge and experiences over various time periods ranging from minutes to years. Retrieval of information from long-term memory occurs in two stages: search and reconstruction.[20] The search stage involves locating the target information. It is then interpreted and reconstructed according to prior knowledge and experiences.

Tulving[21] has differentiated between two aspects of long-term memory: semantic and episodic. Semantic memory, memory for knowledge, is acquired independent of the situational context. For example, most people know that Washington, D.C., is the capital of the United States, but most cannot recall when this information was acquired. Episodic memory is dependent on specific situations and events and allows one to remember past experiences. For example, remembering the people present and the gifts received at a birthday celebration is considered episodic memory. Semantic and episodic memory are not distinct entities but function as an integrated long-term memory system.[20]

Another aspect of long-term memory is the distinction between procedural and declarative memory.[8] Procedural memory is the ability to automatically perform the sequences of a task such as driving a car or operating the videocassette recorder. Individuals may not remember having ever performed such tasks and may be unable to describe the steps involved. However, they may be able to perform the tasks. Declarative memory requires conscious awareness. The individual must be able to specifically explain the event or task.

Semantics/Pragmatics

Language is a complex process involving the comprehension, integration, and expression of an organized set of symbols used for communication.[22] It has been divided into five levels: phonology, morphology, syntax, semantics, and pragmatics. Since semantics and pragmatics are the two levels of language that are primarily affected in the TBI population,[23–25] only these areas will be discussed.

The function of the semantic level of language is to attach meaning to words and sentences. It permits the differentiation between the literal meaning of the sentence and the intended meaning of the speaker.[26] Pragmatic skills are also important in interpreting the speaker's intent. "Pragmatics is the study of the relationships between language behavior and the contexts in which it is used."[27(p1)] Davis and Wilcox[27] consider these contexts to include the physical and social situations and the knowledge, opinions, and emotions of the participants.

Pragmatics is concerned with how the speaker manipulates both the nonverbal and verbal aspects of a message within a particular context to express a desired intention.[28] Nonverbal communication behaviors can augment verbal communication or convey meaning independent of words. These behaviors include eye contact, gestures, body posture and position (proxemics), facial expression, and vocal inflection (prosody).[29] Verbal aspects encompass conversational skills and use of cohesive ties.

Conversational skills include the appropriate initiation of a conversation, introduction of a new topic, maintenance of a topic, and turn-taking skills. Effective conversational skills rely heavily on the adequate comprehension and production of nonverbal behaviors. Cohesive ties, such as reference, substitution, ellipsis, conjunction, and lexical cohesion, allow for a smooth and logical flow of discourse[30] and are important for conversational skills (particularly topic maintenance). Referencing skills include the use of pronouns, demonstratives, or comparatives to refer to previously mentioned items in the text. Similarly, substitution is the use of items of the same grammatical class to refer to previously cited information. In lexical cohesion, a common vocabulary item such as a synonym or superordinate is used to connect the cohesive item and its referent. Ellipsis is the deletion of known information that is shared by the participants. Conjunctions are cohesive devices that relate one clause to another.

COMMUNICATIVE AND EXECUTIVE SYSTEMS

The complex, reciprocal interrelationships among the cognitive and linguistic processes defined previously constitute an integrated unit. This unit interfaces with the output mode to achieve effective overall communicative functioning. The output mode refers to the individual's response system and is affected by neurophysiological factors. For example, if a patient is unable to use the upper extremities due to paralysis, then the ability to gesture is impaired. Similarly, the patient with oral-motor problems is likely to have impaired speech. Although effective communication is dependent in part on the integrity of the available output modes, the focus of this discussion is on the cognitive and linguistic processes that underlie effective communication. Therefore, the output mode is not depicted in Figure 3-1.

The executive system, the central regulatory mechanism, ". . . is involved in setting goals, assessing strengths and weaknesses within the system, planning and directing activity, initiating and inhibiting behavior, monitoring current activity, and evaluating results."[13(p102)] These functions are of prime importance in the self-evaluation and self-monitoring of behavior and contribute to socially appropriate behavior.[13,31] The executive system is considered to be a function of the frontal lobes.[7] It relies on verbal mediation.[7] Therefore, there is a strong interrelationship between the executive and communicative systems. Neither the executive system[1] or the communicative system is a unitary process; rather, they function in combination with each of the other cognitive and linguistic processes to maximize performance.

TREATMENT FRAMEWORK

Figure 3-1 depicts the overall complex relationships among all the cognitive and linguistic processes discussed previously. Included in the box are those processes that may underlie the problems in effective communication and executive functions. Clinical experience has shown that improvements in one process often impact on other processes. Arrows indicate which process might affect another. Treatment is directly focused toward the processes within the box so that effective communication and executive functions can be achieved.

Other researchers[1-5] concur that treatment directed toward the source of the problem is more effective than treating the symptom itself. For ex-

ample, the patient who is unable to read beyond the simple sentence level may not have difficulty with the actual understanding of the printed word but rather difficulty attending to or retaining more lengthy material. Therefore, treatment should be directed toward improving the underlying impaired processes of attention and memory rather than the linguistic component of reading. Another example is the patient who cannot retell a short story. If the difficulty arises from problems in remembering the content of the story, then treatment should be directed toward providing strategies to improve recall. However, if the difficulty arises from problems in organizing the sequence of events in a cohesive manner for expression, the treatment should focus on improving organization skills for discourse.

Discussion of the interrelationships among processes begins with attention. *Attention* is of prime importance because it affects all levels of cognitive processing. A basic level of *alertness/arousal* is needed so that meaningful *perceptions* can be developed from the *sensory reception* of stimuli. Since the basic level of alertness/arousal is determined by physiological factors, it cannot be treated directly. Therefore, sensory stimulation techniques are used as a means of facilitating increased alertness and arousal and subsequently improved perception.

Perception is dependent on focused, sustained, and selective *attention*. These attentional skills allow individuals to filter out irrelevant sensory stimuli and attend to the relevant stimuli long enough to interpret them. Conversely, changes in perception can facilitate improved attentional skills: it is easier to sustain attention to information that has meaning. These same levels of attention and the ability to form meaningful perceptions are necessary for intact *orientation* to person, place, situation, and time.[9]

The complex, higher level cognitive processes of *organization*, *reasoning*, and *problem solving/judgment* require *attention* to multiple pieces of information that are continually manipulated, evaluated, and modified. Therefore, the ability to focus on more than one piece of information at a time, to shift attention from one aspect of the information to another, and the ability to sustain attention over time is crucial. The ability to organize and structure a task will also enable one to sustain, shift, and divide attention more appropriately.

Perception also influences these higher level processes. If perceptions are faulty, these cognitive manipulations will result in inaccurate solutions and conclusions. Conversely, organizational skills can enhance perception by sorting items into familiar classes and grouping related information. This serves to simplify the vast amount of information in the environment.[32]

The abilities to attach meaning to words *(semantics)* and to use language appropriately *(pragmatics)* rely on accurate *perceptions* of and *orientation* to the communicative situation. Communicative interactions cannot occur unless the individual perceives the verbal message and the subtle nonverbal signals given by others. In addition, orientation to the roles of the other participants and the context within which the conversation is taking place is necessary in order to interpret the message appropriately.

Semantics and *pragmatics* are dependent on *organizational* skills. The ability to sequence ideas and events will facilitate the production of discourse that is meaningful, well-ordered, logical, and relevant. An organized content also permits the appropriate use of cohesive ties which then serve to enhance the discourse. *Problem solving/judgment* and *reasoning* also influence the semantic and pragmatic levels of language. Word choice and socially appropriate language behavior will depend on the individual's analysis and judgment of the participants and the situation. Conversely, problem solving/judgment as well as organization and reasoning require semantic and pragmatic skills. An individual must draw upon the semantic content and pragmatic knowledge of the situation in order to sequence information properly, make reasonable inferences, develop logical solutions, and form appropriate opinions.

Memory skills are basic to the adequate functioning of all other cognitive and linguistic processes. The sensory level of memory is important for the integration of sensory information and the formation of meaningful *perceptions*.[33] *Orientation* to person, place, situation, and time requires the pairing of present stimuli in the environment with those retrieved from long-term memory. For example, in order to recognize a person, salient visual and auditory characteristics are identified and compared to information stored in memory.

Attention and *memory* are closely related. For effective attention, both the task requirements and the specific content must be held in working memory. In reverse, all levels of attention are important for maximizing successful encoding to or retrieval from memory. For instance, in order to retrieve information from long-term memory, attention is divided between information in consciousness and that which is stored. Further, attention must be shifted from the search stage to the reconstructive stage of retrieval. The accurate *perceptual* interpretation of sensory stimuli is also necessary for the encoding of information.

Performance of *organizational*, *reasoning*, and *problem solving/judgment* tasks requires that information be temporarily stored in short-term memory. In addition, information that is stored in long-term memory must be retrieved to develop and use organizational strategies, make inferences, draw conclusions, and formulate possible solutions. Reed[32] has discussed how memory specifically impacts on problem solving. First, alternate solutions to a problem are stored in short-term memory for evaluation. Second, long-term memory stores information about prior problem solving experiences and strategies used to attempt to solve them. By recalling these strategies, previous mistakes can be prevented. Finally, the correct problem solving strategy must be stored in long-term memory to facilitate the solving of similar future problems.

Memory also affects *semantics* and *pragmatics*. Comprehension of the meaning of words and sentences is more rapidly achieved when they can be compared to similar concepts available in short- or long-term memory.[32] Prior experience is also important in determining which semantic and pragmatic components may be appropriate to a particular situation so that communication can be more effective.

Semantics, *pragmatics*, *organization*, and *problem solving/judgment* skills are important to *memory*. Systematic storage in and retrieval of information from long-term memory can be facilitated by organizing information according to its meaning. This semantic organization also permits information to be retrieved more rapidly.[32]

CONCLUSION

In summary, this framework is based on the premise that communication and executive functions are impaired in the traumatic brain injured individual primarily because of deficits in any of the processes of sensory reception, attention, perception, orientation, organization, reasoning, problem solving/judgment, semantics, pragmat-ics, and/or memory. The speech-language pathologist who is responsible for the rehabilitation of communication disorders in the traumatic brain injured individual should have an understanding of the factors that could potentially contribute to problems in a specific language modality. The clinical implications for diagnosis and treatment based on this framework are presented in Chapters 4 and 5.

REFERENCES

1. Sohlberg MM, Mateer C. *Introduction to Cognitive Rehabilitation.* New York, NY: Guilford Press; 1989.

2. Bracy OL. Cognitive rehabilitation: a process approach. *Cog Rehabil.* 1986;4:10–17.

3. Ben-Yishay Y, Diller L. Cognitive deficits. In: Rosenthal M, Griffith ER, Bond MR, Miller JD, eds. *Rehabilitation of the Head Injured Adult.* Philadelphia, Pa: FA Davis Co; 1983:167–183.

4. Ben-Yishay Y, Diller L. Cognitive remediation. In: Rosenthal M, Griffith ER, Bond MR, Miller JD, eds. *Rehabilitation of the Head Injured Adult.* Philadelphia, Pa: FA Davis; 1983:367–380.

5. Hagen C. Language disorders secondary to closed head injury: diagnosis and treatment. *Top Lang Disord.* 1981;1:73–87.

6. Mesulam MM. Attention, confusional states, and neglect. In: Mesulam MM, ed. *Principles of Behavioral Neurology.* Philadelphia, Pa: FA Davis Co; 1985:125–168.

7. Luria AR. *The Working Brain: An Introduction to Neuropsychology.* New York, NY: Basic Books; 1973.

8. Sohlberg MM, Mateer CA. Effectiveness of an attention training program. *J Clin Exper Neuropsych.* 1987;9:117–130.

9. Lezak M. *Neuropsychological Assessment.* 2nd ed. New York, NY: Oxford University Press; 1983.

10. Gibson EJ. *Principles of Perceptual Learning and Development.* New York, NY: Appleton-Century-Crofts; 1969.

11. Mesulam MM. Patterns in behavioral neuroanatomy: association areas, the limbic system, and hemispheric specialization. In: Mesulam MM, ed. *Principles of Behavioral Neurology.* Philadelphia, Pa: FA Davis; 1985:1–70.

12. Strub RL, Black FW. *The Mental Status Examination in Neurology.* Philadelphia, Pa: FA Davis Co; 1977.

13. Szekeres SF, Ylvisaker M, Cohen SB. A framework for cognitive rehabilitation therapy. In: Ylvisaker M, Gobble EMR, eds. *Community Re-entry for Head Injured Adults.* Boston, Mass: College-Hill Press; 1987:87–136.

14. Luria AR. *Human Brain and Psychological Processes.* New York, NY: Harper and Row; 1966.

15. Baddeley AD. Memory theory and memory therapy. In: Wilson BA, Moffat N, eds. *Clinical Management of Memory Problems.* Gaithersburg, Md: Aspen Publishers Inc; 1984:5–27.

16. Atkinson RC, Shiffrin R. Human memory: a proposed system and its control processes. In: Spence KW, Spence JT, eds. *The Psychology of Learning and Motivation: Advances in Research and Theory.* New York, NY: Academic Press; 1968;2:89–195.

17. Squire LR. *Memory and Brain.* New York, NY: Oxford University Press; 1987.

18. Baddeley AD, Hitch GJ. Working memory. In: Bower GA, ed. *The Psychology of Learning and Motivation: Advances in Research and Theory.* New York, NY: Academic Press; 1974;8:47–90.

19. Monsell S. Components of working memory underlying verbal skills: a "distributed capacities" view. In: Bouma H, Bouwhuis D, eds. *International Symposium on Attention and Performance.* Hillsdale, NJ: Erlbaum; 1984;10:327–350.

20. Rumelhart DE. *Introduction to Human Information Processing.* New York, NY: John Wiley and Sons; 1977.

21. Tulving E. Episodic and semantic memory. In: Tulving E, Donaldson W, eds. *Organization of Memory.* New York, NY: Academic Press; 1972:381–403.

22. Nicolosi L, Harryman E, Kresheck J. *Terminology of Communication Disorders: Speech, Language, Hearing.* Baltimore, Md: Williams and Wilkins Co; 1978.

23. Mentis M, Prutting CA. Cohesion in the discourse of normal and head-injured adults. *J Speech Hear Res.* 1987;30:88–90.

24. Milton SB, Prutting CA, Binder GM. Appraisal of communicative competence in head injured adults. In: Brookshire RH, ed. *Clinical Aphasiology Conference Proceedings.* Minneapolis, Minn: BRK Publishers; 1984:114–123.

25. Holland AL. When is aphasia aphasia? the problem of closed head injury. In: Brookshire RH, ed. *Clinical Aphasiology Conference Proceedings.* Minneapolis, Minn: BRK Publishers; 1982:345–349.

26. Bayles KA, Kasniak AW. *Communication and Cognition in Normal Aging and Dementia.* Boston, Mass: College-Hill Press; 1987.

27. Davis GA, Wilcox MJ. *Adult Aphasia Rehabilitation: Applied Pragmatics.* San Diego, Calif: College-Hill Press; 1985.

28. Burns MS. Language without communication: the pragmatics of right hemisphere damage. In: Burns MS, Halper AS, Mogil SI. *Clinical Management of Right Hemisphere Dysfunction.* Gaithersburg, Md: Aspen Publishers Inc; 1985:17–28.

29. Burns MS, Halper AS, Mogil SI. Diagnosis of communication problems in right hemisphere damage. In: Burns MS, Halper AS, Mogil SI. *Clinical Management of Right Hemisphere Dysfunction.* Gaithersburg, Md: Aspen Publishers Inc; 1985:29–38.

30. Halliday MAK, Hassan R. *Cohesion in English.* London: Longman; 1976.

31. Ylvisaker M, Szekeres S. Metacognitive and executive impairments in head-injured children and adults. *Top Lang Disord.* 1989;9:34–49.

32. Reed SK. *Cognition: Theory and Applications.* Monterey, Calif: Brooks/Cole Publishing Co; 1982.

33. Wilson BA. *Rehabilitation of Memory.* New York, NY: Guilford Press; 1987.

Chapter 4

Evaluation of Communication Problems in the Traumatic Brain Injured Adult

Trudy K. Miller, Anita S. Halper, and Leora R. Cherney

The evaluation of patients with traumatic brain injury involves determining which individual processes described in Chapter 3 are impaired, the potential effects of the impaired processes on one another, and their total impact on communicative and executive functions. The purpose of this chapter is to present guidelines for such an assessment. The evaluation of aphasia, dysarthria, and dysphagia is not addressed as assessment procedures for these diagnoses are available elsewhere.[1-9]

The assessment of patients with TBI should allow the speech-language pathologist to: (1) make an accurate differential diagnosis of the communication disorder; (2) identify the patient's strengths and weaknesses; (3) establish pretreatment baseline measures for later measurement of recovery; (4) develop an individualized treatment plan with long- and short-term goals; (5) determine a prognosis; and (6) define a plan for family counseling.[10,11]

Recently a number of tools have become available for use with the TBI adult (see Appendix 4-A). However, rarely does one single tool adequately evaluate all the cognitive and linguistic processes described in Chapter 3.

The tools selected for assessment vary in part according to the level of the patient. Hagen and Malkmus have developed a tool for identifying patients' "Levels of Cognitive Functioning" (LOCF).[12] It delineates eight stages in the recovery of cognitive functioning and describes the associated linguistic components at each stage (see Table 4-1). This tool was developed as a behavior rating scale to assist in the evaluation of the traumatic brain injured patient. However, we have found it more useful clinically to divide patients into two main levels according to the degree to which they can actively participate in the evaluation process. The approach to the patient, the focus of the evaluation, and the type of tests used will differ accordingly.

Level 1 patients are the most severely involved. They display reduced alertness/arousal and responsiveness to the environment and are nonparticipatory in a test situation. This level corresponds to Levels I–III of the LOCF. Only an informal assessment can be accomplished with

Table 4-1 Levels of Cognitive Functioning and Expected Behaviors

	Response Type	Description
Level I	No response	Unresponsive to all stimuli
Level II	Generalized response	Inconsistent, nonpurposeful, nonspecific reactions to stimuli; responds to pain, but response may be delayed
Level III	Localized response	Inconsistent reaction directly related to type of stimulus presented; responds to some commands; may respond to discomfort
Level IV	Confused, agitated response	Disoriented and unaware of present events with frequent bizarre and inappropriate behavior; attention span is short and ability to process information is impaired
Level V	Confused, inappropriate, nonagitated response	Nonpurposeful, random or fragmented responses when task complexity exceeds abilities; patient appears alert and responds to simple commands; performs previously learned tasks but is unable to learn new ones
Level VI	Confused, appropriate response	Behavior is goal-directed; responses are appropriate to the situation with incorrect responses because of memory difficulties
Level VII	Automatic, appropriate response	Correct routine responses that are robot-like; appears oriented to setting, but insight, judgment, and problem solving are poor
Level VIII	Purposeful, appropriate response	Correct responding, carryover of new learning; no required supervision, poor tolerance for stress, and some abstract reasoning difficulties.

Source: Hagen C, Malkmus D. Intervention strategies for language disorders secondary to head trauma. Presented at the American Speech-Language-Hearing Association Annual Convention; 1979; Atlanta, Ga.

these patients. The evaluation focuses on determining the patient's degree of responsiveness to a variety of sensory stimuli.

Level 2, a broad category, corresponds to Levels IV–VIII of the LOCF. It includes patients who have the potential to actively participate in the evaluation process. The evaluation now focuses on identifying the cognitive and linguistic processes that are impaired. Both informal and formal tests typically are used with Level 2 patients at the lower (more impaired) end of the continuum of severity. Primarily formal measures are administered to patients at the higher (less impaired) end of the continuum. Further, selection of these tests should take into consideration the patient's premorbid educational, vocational, and avocational status.

ASSESSMENT GUIDELINES FOR LEVEL 1 PATIENTS

Patients at Level 1 may occasionally respond to stimuli but with movements that are nonpurposeful and delayed. Prior to assessment, the speech-language pathologist should determine the patient's most responsive times of day by talking with family members and nursing staff. The evaluation should then be conducted at these times. Initially the clinician should note the patient's physical and medical status, including typical and abnormal postures and the presence of respiratory and nutritional supports. The clinician should then observe the patient's wakefulness and responsiveness to stimuli that occur naturally in the environment. Finally, stimuli should be presented via all sensory channels (i.e., auditory, visual, olfactory, gustatory, and tactile) to determine those stimuli to which the patient is most responsive. The type, consistency, and latency of the patient's responses to this stimulation should be noted. The patient's behavior with and without sensory stimulation should be compared so that responsiveness to the specific stimuli can be identified.

A quick but gross measure of level of consciousness is the Glasgow Coma Scale.[13,14] It assesses three areas: eye opening; the best motor response; and verbal response (see Table 4-2). Scores may range from 3 to 15. According to the authors of the scale, a score of nine or more indicates that the patient is out of coma. However, we feel that many patients with a score lower than nine might be appropriate for a sensory stimulation program. It is important to look at the type of response exhibited within each area. For example, a patient with a score of three for eye opening, two for motor response and one for verbal response would be a candidate for a trial period in a sensory stimulation program. The Glasgow Coma Scale can be used on a daily or weekly basis to determine change in level of consciousness.

Stimulus Presentation

It is important that all stimuli be presented in a consistent manner to ensure reliability for subsequent retesting. The speech-language pathologist should observe the patient's responses to nonverbal and verbal auditory stimuli presented at varying volumes. Nonverbal stimuli include environmental sounds, noisemakers, and music. Verbal stimuli include the patient's name, simple one-step commands requiring responses compatible with the patient's physical status, and general conversation. The clinician should determine if there is a differential response to familiar versus unfamiliar voices. The side from which auditory stimuli is presented should be varied to determine whether the patient can localize to a sound source.

The presence of a protective reflex to visual threat, the ability to focus on and track visual stimuli, and the ability to focus and maintain eye contact are assessed. The speech-language pathologist should observe for a protective eye blink to objects that are moved rapidly toward the eye. Response to light such as turning on a flashlight in a darkened room or switching room lights on and

Table 4-2 Glasgow Coma Scale

		Response	*Score*
Eyes	Open	Spontaneously	4
		To verbal command	3
		To pain	2
		No response	1
Best Motor Response	To verbal commands	Obeys	6
	To painful stimuli	Localizes pain	5
		Flexion, withdrawal	4
		Flexion, abnormal (decerebrate rigidity)	3
		Extension (decerebrate rigidity)	2
		No response	1
Best Verbal Response		Oriented and converses	5
		Disoriented and converses	4
		Inappropriate words	3
		Incomprehensible sounds	2
		No response	1

off should be noted. Brightly colored objects and pictures can be presented to evaluate the ability to focus visual gaze. To assess visual tracking skills a flashlight, brightly colored objects, or pictures can be moved across the patient's visual field.

The patient's response to a variety of olfactory, gustatory, and/or tactile stimuli should be observed. To assess the olfactory and gustatory channels, both noxious and pleasant stimuli are presented. Noxious stimuli are disagreeable to a patient and depend on personal likes and dislikes. Noxious scents might include rubbing alcohol, garlic, and vinegar while pleasant scents might include vanilla and banana extract or familiar colognes. A variety of fruit juices placed on the lips, tongue, and/or gums can be used to assess response to pleasant tastes; onion and lemon concentrates are used as noxious stimuli. Cagan[15] has indicated that individuals are more apt to respond to bitter tastes than sweet, sour, or salty.

Tactile stimuli should be applied to the hands, arms, face, and oral motor structures including the lips, gums, teeth, and cheeks. The patient's response to light touch (e.g., feathers, gentle stroking) and deep pressure (e.g., massage) should be observed. The clinician should note whether the patient responds differentially to hot versus cold, slow versus quick, and smooth (e.g., satin) versus rough (e.g., sandpaper) stimulation.

Response Measurement

Patient responses can be categorized according to the following seven point scale:

6 = consistent related localized response
5 = consistent unrelated localized response
4 = inconsistent related localized response
3 = inconsistent unrelated localized response
2 = consistent generalized response
1 = inconsistent generalized response
0 = no response

A consistent response is one that occurs after every presentation of a specific sensory stimulus while an inconsistent response occurs only periodically. A related response is directly associated with the type of stimulus presented whereas an unrelated response has no direct association with the stimulus. In some patients a related response may not be possible because of physical limitations. A localized response is one that is confined to a particular area of the body that is close to where the specific sensory stimulus is applied. On the other hand, a generalized response may involve more than one part of the body or be geographically distant from the point of stimulation See Table 4-3 for examples.

The type of response elicited may vary depending on the specific stimuli and/or the physiological status of the patient at the time of the evaluation. The clinician should observe for any of the following responses:

- change in skin color and temperature/sweating
- change in respiratory rate, either a slowing or a quickening
- increase or decrease in general muscle tone
- movement of the body
- change in facial expression
- eye blinking/eye movements
- oral-motor responses (e.g., suckle-swallow, biting)
- vocalizations

Table 4-3 Categorizing Patient Responses

Stimulus	Response	Rating
Ringing bells	Startle	Generalized
	Eye blink	Unrelated localized
	Turning head to sound source	Related localized
Q-tip dipped in juice applied to tongue	Increased respiratory rate	Generalized
	Head turn	Unrelated localized
	Suckle	Related localized

The Western Neuro Sensory Stimulation Profile

An alternative to the evaluation guidelines described above is the Western Neuro Sensory Stimulation Profile (WNSSP).[16] It was designed to objectively measure cognitive/communicative functioning in TBI patients with a LOCF of II, III, IV, and early stages of level V. Reliability and validity of the test have been established. This test is appropriate for our Level 1 patients and those Level 2 patients at the lower end of the severity continuum.

The WNSSP consists of 33 items which assess arousal/attention, expressive communication, and response to auditory, visual, tactile, and olfactory stimulation. The items are scored using a multi-point system which provides a mechanism for obtaining more objective scores. However, the point system varies from item to item making it cumbersome and time consuming for the speech-language pathologist to score. Therefore, we prefer using our seven point scale for Level 1 patients.

ASSESSMENT GUIDELINES FOR LEVEL 2 PATIENTS

Level 2 patients at the lower end of the continuum of severity are beginning to use language appropriately. Although they are able to participate in limited formal testing, their attention is brief and they are easily distracted. Patients in the middle range of the severity continuum communicate appropriately in simple familiar contexts, but behavioral and cognitive problems are conspicuous. They can attend to testing but may be distracted by the environment and require redirection to the task. Patients at the upper end of the range can communicate appropriately in a variety of contexts. Their cognitive deficits are subtle; difficulties in shifting and divided attention may interfere with testing.

Informal and formal evaluation tasks requiring different cognitive and linguistic processes should be administered. An analysis of the processes involved in each task allows the speech-language pathologist to determine the possible underlying cause of the patient's errors on that task. Then, an analysis of the trends in performance across different tasks should be conducted to more precisely identify the impaired processes. Sohlberg and Mateer[17] have referred to this as a process specific approach to the assessment of cognitive-linguistic functions. Throughout both informal and formal assessment, the speech-language pathologist should observe functions of the executive system including the patient's ability to recognize errors, self-correct, self-monitor and inhibit behavior, and plan activities.

Screening

The first step in the evaluation of Level 2 patients should be a screening. The purpose is to tentatively determine which cognitive and linguistic processes seem to affect the overall effectiveness of communicative and executive functions. These processes will then be the focus of further evaluation; appropriate informal and/or formal assessment tools will be chosen accordingly.

It has been our experience that certain subtests of the Boston Diagnostic Aphasia Examination (BDAE)[1] serve as an appropriate screening tool for TBI patients. While some patients will not be able to perform all of the suggested subtests, the pattern of performance and the successes and failures further guide the direction of the evaluation. Although the BDAE has been designed and standardized for persons with aphasia, a qualitative analysis of the TBI patient's performance will provide information about the disrupted processes affecting the communication and executive systems. A quantitative score is also useful in comparing initial, interim, and discharge status to assess progress. Raw scores or percentages should be used rather than the percentile scores that have been derived from normative data on aphasic patients.

Table 4-4 lists the subtests of the BDAE that are recommended as a screening tool and the cognitive and linguistic processes that underlie each task. These subtests are quick and easy to administer, address all language modalities, and tap all the cognitive and linguistic processes except problem solving. Informal measures of problem solving ability can be utilized to augment the screening, if

Table 4-4 Boston Diagnostic Aphasia Examination: Selected Subtests for Screening

Subtest	Cognitive/Linguistic Process
Commands	Memory, Semantics
Complex Ideational Material	Memory, Semantics, Reasoning
Conversation and Expository Speech	Semantics, Pragmatics, Visual Perception, Organization
Repeating Phrases	Attention, Memory, Auditory Perception
Responsive Naming	Attention, Semantics
Animal Naming	Semantics, Organization, Reasoning (Divergent)
Oral Sentence Reading	Attention, Visual Perception
Comprehension of Oral Spelling	Attention, Auditory Perception, Memory
Reading Sentences and Paragraphs	Visual Perception, Semantics, Reasoning
Spelling to Dictation	Semantics, Memory
Narrative Writing	Visual Perception, Semantics, Organization
Sentences Written to Dictation	Semantics, Memory

necessary, and are described later in this chapter. The suggested BDAE subtests also identify those TBI patients with aphasia (e.g., Wernicke's, Broca's) or a specific aphasic component (e.g., word retrieval problems). It should be remembered that attention is a prerequisite for performing any task. Therefore, in Table 4-4 this process is noted only when the subtest is particularly useful for assessing attention.

A research edition of a screening test for TBI is available. The Brief Test of Head Injury (BTHI)[18] is designed to probe the following: orientation/attention; following one to three step commands; linguistic organization including seriation, categorization, differences, analogies, sequencing, and picture description; reading comprehension of words and sentences; object and picture naming; immediate, short- and long-term memory; and visual-spatial skills including matching and recall. It allows for the patient who is unable to respond verbally to receive full credit for nonverbal responses. The test can be administered within 25–30 minutes and is particularly useful in establishing baseline behaviors and tracking recovery.

The BTHI is most appropriate for screening those Level 2 patients at the lower end of the severity continuum. Within our framework, it directly probes the cognitive and linguistic processes of attention, perception, orientation, memory, semantics, and organization. In addition, the speech-language pathologist can interpret the patient's pragmatic behaviors from the initial interview portion of the test.

Informal Observations

Informal assessment procedures tap each process in a more functional setting and can be performed not only in the treatment room but in a more natural environment. They can be tailored to the patient's specific needs and premorbid interests. The flexibility of informal testing allows the clinician to manipulate cues and identify those which maximize the patient's performance. Although the testing is informally administered, it is important to present the stimuli in a consistent format. Responses should also be measured and documented in the same way at each administration. This permits the clinician to more objectively assess progress. Sohlberg and Mateer[17] have presented a rating scale, the Good Samaritan Hospital's Cognitive Behavioral Rating Scale, which may assist in documenting observations of patients' functional performance. This scale outlines four levels of performance in each of the processes of attention/concentration, memory, visual processing, reasoning/problem solving, executive functions, and language.

Attention

During conversation, the clinician should observe the patient's ability to focus and sustain attention to the speaker and the topic. Further, the patient's ability to sustain attention while performing a variety of informal and formal tasks should be determined. The speech-language pathologist should measure the length of time the patient sustains attention to a task, the ease with which the patient can be redirected back to the task, and the types and number of cues necessary. If there is a discrepancy between sustaining attention to auditory or visual stimuli, this should also be noted.

Selective attention can be assessed by observing the patient's ability to focus and sustain attention to the target stimuli while ignoring extraneous external stimuli in a distracting environment. The clinician should differentiate the extent to which the patient is distracted by external stimuli within the environment and/or internal stimuli which are self-generated. Informal vigilance tasks that require the patient to respond to a target stimulus embedded within a series of other stimuli (e.g., every time you see or hear the word yellow, raise your hand) evaluates both sustained and selective attention.

Alternating or shifting attention can be assessed by ascertaining the ease with which the patient shifts from one subtest to another subtest with different task requirements. The type and number of cues required to shift attention also should be noted. Divided attention is typically assessed through functional tasks such as listening to a lecture while simultaneously taking notes or talking on the telephone while opening mail.

Perception

All patients should have a standard pure tone evaluation of hearing acuity to rule out hearing loss that may be contributing to an auditory problem. Difficulty understanding simple commands and basic conversation may be present despite adequate hearing acuity, attention, and short-term memory. Then, formal measures of auditory perception and central auditory processing testing may be indicated.

The presence of visual acuity deficits should be ruled out before proceeding with visual perceptual testing. Typically, this information is obtained from the patient's medical chart or from the physician. Informal visual perceptual testing may be indicated for patients with a significantly reduced attention span and difficulty following multiple directions. The clinician should have the patient read aloud a short passage or copy a sentence and observe for evidence of left-sided neglect, tracking and scanning problems, and visual-spatial deficits. The patient may omit or misread words, omit words only on the left or right side of the page, skip lines, or be unable to shift from the end of one line to the beginning of the next line.

Orientation

The speech-language pathologist relies on family and hospital staff reports as well as observations of the patient in functional settings to assess recognition of persons. The patient's response to familiar persons and new acquaintances, such as the clinician, should be noted. Orientation to place includes evaluating the patient's awareness of the present location and the ability to move independently around familiar and less familiar surroundings. Orientation to situation is determined by asking patients about their present condition and the circumstances leading up to it. Knowledge of time concepts and the ability to monitor the passage of time should be assessed. This includes telling time, providing the day, date, year, and season as well as estimating how long a period of time has elapsed or how long a specific activity will take. It is important to note how effectively the patient is able to use clinician- or self-generated environmental cues.

Semantics/Pragmatics

The speech-language pathologist should evaluate whether the vocabulary level of the patient is consistent with premorbid status. Evidence of word finding problems such as inappropriate pauses, circumlocutions, and verbal paraphasias should be noted. Difficulty comprehending conversation may also be a symptom of semantic problems. Formal testing can be utilized to corroborate these observations.

The effectiveness of the patient's pragmatic skills should be assessed through conversation in different situations (e.g., talking to the physician, chatting with other patients, ordering food in the cafeteria). Signs of difficulty in the appropriate use of gestures and intonation, turn-taking skills, topic initiation and maintenance, and organization and completeness of discourse should be documented. Rating scales are available to provide structure to the evaluation of pragmatics.[19-22] Exhibit 4-1, the RICE Rating Scale of Pragmatic Communication Skills,[20] is an example of one of these scales.

Organization/Reasoning/Problem Solving

Most testing for these higher level cognitive processes is formal. However, in addition to the required response on the formal test, it is often helpful for the patient to explain the reason for the response given. This may assist the clinician in determining whether a specific strategy was used and in evaluating its effectiveness. The patient's ability to sequence the day's events or the steps in a task, formulate alternate solutions to an emergency situation, and form an opinion about a person in the news also can be assessed informally.

Memory

Memory can be informally assessed by reviewing orientation information and then questioning for retention. At the end of a session, the speech-language pathologist may question the patient regarding events of the session and other pertinent activities of the day. The patient's recall of auditorily or visually presented information should be investigated as well as knowledge of recent and remote biographical and historical information. When interpreting the results, the clinician should be aware that the various components of memory may be affected differentially.

Formal Testing

Appendix 4-A is an annotated list of formal standardized tests. While this list is not exhaustive, it includes those tests or selected subtests that we have found to be the most valuable for assessing the cognitive-linguistic skills of the TBI adult. The appendix indicates the severity of the patient for which each test/subtest is appropriate. Listed are those processes that are primarily assessed by the test, although several other processes may be required to perform the task. The speech-language pathologist should consider these other processes in analyzing the reasons for the patient's difficulty with the task. For example, a patient may have problems performing a reasoning task that is presented visually, because of visual-perceptual deficits rather than reasoning deficits. Failure also could be the result of attentional problems, because attention is a prerequisite for performing any task. Many of the test items are complex and may require more processes than indicated by the stated purpose of the test. Information about normative data or ways to interpret the test results when the norms are not appropriate for the adult TBI population are provided.

Appendix 4-A is helpful in the selection of an appropriate test battery. The test battery will vary for each patient depending on the following factors: severity level of the patient; the impaired cognitive and linguistic processes identified from the screening; the patient's premorbid educational, vocational, and avocational status; the patient/ family goals; and the normative data provided by the test.

Listed in Appendix 4-B are academic achievement tests that are highly dependent on language skills. These provide supplementary information for determining potential school or vocational placement and should be administered at the appropriate stage of rehabilitation. These tests would not be used to specifically assess cognitive and linguistic processes. Information about normative data is provided. Those patients who exceed the age and educational levels of the test norms would be expected to score at the highest level.

Exhibit 4-1 The RICE Rating Scale of Pragmatic Communication Skills

A. Nonverbal Communication

	1	2	3	4	5
Intonation	Flat or stereotyped		Limited or inappropriate		Appropriate
Facial Expression	None		Limited or inappropriate		Appropriate
Eye Contact	Cannot establish or maintain eye contact		Needs cues to establish or maintain eye contact		Appropriate
Gestures and Proxemics	Inappropriate or does not use		Inconsistent appropriate use		Appropriate

B. Conversational Skills

	1	2	3	4	5
Conversational Initiation	Inappropriate or does not initiate		Inconsistent appropriate initiation		Appropriate
Turn-taking	Does not obey signals		Inconsistently responsive to signals		Adequate
Verbosity	Over 50% of responses are verbose or tangential		25% to 50% of responses are verbose or tangential		Appropriate response length

C. Use of Linguistic Context

	1	2	3	4	5
Topic Maintenance	Maintains topic less than 25% of the time		Maintains topic 50% of the time		Maintains topic
Presupposition	Presupposes too much and/or too little 50%		Presupposes too much and/or too little 25% to 50%		Appropriate
Referencing Skills	Inappropriate referencing		Inconsistent appropriate referencing		Appropriate

D. Organization of a Narrative

	1	2	3	4	5
Organization	Disorganized		Some organization but lacks a unifying theme		Adequate
Completeness	More than 50% of details are missing and/or inaccurate		25% to 50% of details are missing or inaccurate		Adequate

Source: Reprinted from *Clinical Management of Right Hemisphere Dysfunction* (pp 50–51) by MS Burns, AS Halper and SI Mogil, Aspen Publishers, Inc, © 1985.

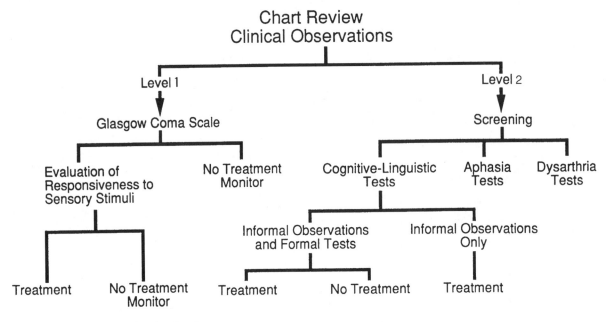

Figure 4-1 Steps in the Evaluation Process

CONCLUSION

Figure 4-1 summarizes the steps involved in the evaluation of patients with traumatic brain injury. First, the speech-language pathologist determines whether the patient falls in the Level 1 or 2 category through chart review and preliminary observations.

For Level 1 patients, the Glasgow Coma Scale[13,14] can be administered. Based on a quantitative score and a qualitative analysis of the patient's responses, a decision can be made about the need for further evaluation of responsiveness to sensory stimuli. If not indicated, the patient should be monitored periodically to determine if any change has occurred. If further evaluation of responsiveness to stimuli is appropriate, the clinician can use the guidelines described in this chapter in the section on assessment of Level 1 patients or the Western Neuro Sensory Stimulation Pro-

file.[16] Based on these results, a decision is made regarding candidacy for treatment.

Patients who are categorized as Level 2 are first screened. Their performance on the screening tasks is analyzed to identify the presence of aphasia and/or dysarthria and to tentatively determine which cognitive-linguistic processes are impaired. If an aphasia or a dysarthria is suspected, specific tests designed to evaluate these disorders should be administered. When cognitive-linguistic impairments are suspected, informal observations and/or formal tests are selected to further evaluate these areas. Appendix 4-A can be used as a guide for test selection. It provides information about the processes tapped by each subtest and the severity of the patient for whom it is most appropriate. An analysis of the pattern of impairments in each of the processes allows the speech-language pathologist to design an appropriate treatment program.

REFERENCES

1. Goodglass H, Kaplan E. *The Assessment of Aphasia and Related Language Disorders*. Philadelphia, Pa: Lea and Febiger; 1983.
2. Kertesz A. *Western Aphasia Battery*. New York, NY: Grune and Stratton; 1982.
3. Porch BE. *The Porch Index of Communicative Ability*. Palo Alto, Calif: Consulting Psychologists Press; 1967.
4. Schuell H. *The Minnesota Test for Differential Diagnosis of Aphasia*. Minneapolis, Minn: University of Minnesota Press; 1965.

5. Helm-Estabrooks N, Ramsberger G, Morgan AR, Nicholas M. *BASA: Boston Assessment of Severe Aphasia.* San Antonio, Tex: Special Press; 1989.

6. Darley FL, Aronson AE, Brown JR. *Motor Speech Disorders.* Philadelphia, Pa: WB Saunders Co; 1975.

7. Yorkston KM, Beukelman DR. *Assessment of Intelligibility of Dysarthric Speech.* Tigard, Oreg: CC Publications; 1981.

8. Cherney LR, Cantieri CA, Pannell JJ. *Clinical Evaluation of Dysphagia.* Gaithersburg, Md: Aspen Publishers Inc; 1986.

9. Logemann JA. *Evaluation and Treatment of Swallowing Disorders.* San Diego, Calif: College-Hill Press; 1983.

10. Wolfe G. Clinical neuropsychology and assessment of brain impairment: an overview. *Cog Rehab.* 1987;2:6–9.

11. Baxter R, Cohen SB, Ylvisaker M. Comprehensive cognitive assessment. In: Ylvisaker M, ed. *Head Injury Rehabilitation.* Boston, Mass: College-Hill Press; 1985:247–286.

12. Hagen C, Malkmus D. Intervention strategies for language disorders secondary to head trauma. Presented at the American Speech-Language-Hearing Association Annual Convention; 1979; Atlanta, Ga.

13. Teasdale G, Jennett B. Assessment of coma and impaired consciousness: a practical scale. *Lancet.* 1974;2:81–84.

14. Jennett B, Snoak J, Bond M, Brooks N. Disability after severe head injury: observations on the use of the Glasgow Outcome Scale. *J Neurol, Neurosurg, Psychiatr.* 1981;44:285–293.

15. Cagan RH. Olfaction and gustation: Section B functions and mechanisms. In: Shaw JH, Sweeney EA, Cappuccino CC, Meller SM, eds. *Textbook of Oral Biology.* Philadelphia, Pa: WB Saunders Co; 1978:649–671.

16. Ansell B, Keenan J. *The Western Neuro Sensory Stimulation Profile: A tool for assessing slow-to-recover head-injured patients.* Tustin, Calif: Western Neuro Care Center; 1989.

17. Sohlberg MM, Mateer CA. The assessment of cognitive-communicative functions in head injury. *Topics in Lang Dis.* 1989;9:15–33.

18. Helm-Estabrooks N, Hotz G. *Brief Test of Head Injury: Research Edition Manual.* San Antonio, Tex: Special Press; 1990.

19. Prutting CA, Kirchner DM. A clinical appraisal of the pragmatic aspects of language. *JSHD.* 1987;52:105–119.

20. Burns MS, Halper AS, Mogil SI. Diagnosis of communication problems in right hemisphere damage. In: Burns MS, Halper AS, Mogil SI, eds. *Clinical Management of Right Hemisphere Dysfunction.* Gaithersburg, Md: Aspen Publishers Inc; 1985:29–38.

21. Ehrlich JS, Sipes AL. Group treatment of communication skills for head trauma patients. *Cog Rehab.* 1985;3:32–37.

22. Ehrlich J, Barry P. Rating communication behaviours in the head-injured adult. *Brain Injury.* 1989;3:193–198.

Formal Tests

KEY

Population

LO = Level 2 patients at the lower end of the continuum of severity
MI = Level 2 patients in the middle of the continuum of severity
HI = Level 2 patients at the upper (high) end of the continuum of severity

Process

A = Attention
M = Memory
ORG = Organization
O = Orientation
P = Perception
PR = Pragmatics
PJ = Problem Solving/Judgment
R = Reasoning
S = Semantics

	Population			Process								
	LO	MI	HI	A	M	ORG	O	P	PR	PJ	R	S
The Airplane List by Herbert F. Crovitz. Memory retraining in brain damaged patients; the airplane list. *Cortex*. 1979;15:131–134. Assesses ability to recall a list of 10 words embedded in a passage read aloud. The author of the test indicates that most individuals recall all 10 words in both forward and backward sequence.		✔	✔	✔	✔							
Assessment of Strategies for Auditory Recall (ASAR) by C.S. Brown and G.A. DiCola Forsythe Memorial Hospital, 3333 Silas Creek Parkway, Winston-Salem, NC 27103.												

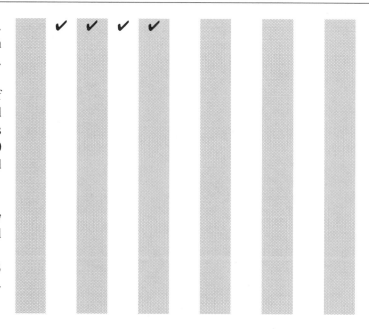

| | Population | | | Process | | | | | | | | |
	LO	MI	HI	A	M	ORG	O	P	PR	PJ	R	S
Orientation Subtest Assesses orientation to person, place, and time	✔	✔			✔		✔					
Sentence Repetition Subtest Assesses immediate recall of sentences		✔		✔	✔							
Paragraph Retention Subtest Assesses recall of lists of related and unrelated words		✔	✔		✔	✔		✔				
Word Retention Subtest Assesses recall of lists of related and unrelated words		✔	✔	✔	✔	✔						

This test was designed primarily to determine whether a patient can benefit from learning a specific treatment protocol for improving memory, the Brown's Listening and Reading Strategies. The authors indicate that if patients fall under the 25th percentile, they are not candidates for this program. Even though we typically do not use Brown's program, the subtests can provide useful information about the cognitive-communicative processes. Norms are provided for individuals aged 17–27 with an average of 13.8 years of education.

Boston Naming Test by Edith Kaplan, Harold Goodglass, and Sandra Weintraub. Lea and Febiger, 600 South Washington Square, Philadelphia, PA 19106.		✔	✔									✔

Assesses ability to name pictures requiring vocabulary of increasing complexity. Mean performance, standard deviation and range are available for normal adults aged 18–59 and for adults with either 12 years

	Population			Process								
	LO	MI	HI	A	M	ORG	O	P	PR	PJ	R	S
or less of education or more than 12 years of education.												
Clinical Evaluation of Language Functions-Revised (CELF-R) by Eleanor Messing Semmel and Elisabeth H. Wiig. The Psychological Corporation, P.O. Box 839954, San Antonio, TX 78283.												
Oral Directions Assesses ability to recall, interpret, and follow oral commands of increasing length and complexity		✔	✔		✔							✔
Formulated Sentences Assesses ability to formulate sentences that include one or two given words		✔	✔									✔
Recalling Sentences Assesses ability to repeat sentences of increasing length and complexity	✔	✔		✔	✔							
Word Classes Assesses ability to identify two of four words that are related semantically, antonymously, spatially, or temporally		✔				✔						✔
Sentence Assembly Assesses ability to sequence words and phrases into sentences		✔				✔						✔
Semantic Relationships Assesses ability to interpret auditorily presented sentences containing temporal, spatial, passive, and comparative relationships		✔			✔							✔
Word Associations Assesses generative naming of		✔	✔									✔

	Population			Process								
	LO	MI	HI	A	M	ORG	O	P	PR	PJ	R	S
animals, transportation, and occupations												
Listening to Paragraphs Assesses interpretation and recall of auditorily presented paragraphs			✔		✔							

Scores are standardized for individuals ages 5-0 through 16-11. For each subtest, raw scores can be converted to standard scores and percentile ranks. An adult with a high school education should score within the normal range for a 16-11 year old.

Detroit Tests of Learning Aptitude (DTLA-2) by Donald D. Hammill. Pro-Ed, 8700 Shoal Creek Blvd., Austin, TX 78758.

	Population			Process								
	LO	MI	HI	A	M	ORG	O	P	PR	PJ	R	S
Subtest II: Sentence Imitation Assesses ability to imitate sentences	✔	✔		✔	✔							
Subtest III: Oral Directions Assesses ability to comprehend and recall directions of increasing complexity		✔	✔		✔							✔
Subtest IV: Word Sequences Assesses ability to auditorily recall a series of unrelated words	✔	✔	✔	✔	✔							
Subtest V: Story Construction Assesses ability to spontaneously produce a story about a given picture	✔	✔	✔						✔			✔
Subtest VI: Design Reproduction Assesses ability to reproduce figures from memory	✔	✔	✔		✔			✔				
Subtest VII: Object Sequences Assesses ability to recall the se-		✔	✔		✔	✔						

| | Population | | | Process | | | | | | | | |
	LO	MI	HI	A	M	ORG	O	P	PR	PJ	R	S
quence of a series of objects from memory												
Subtest VIII: Symbolic Relations Assesses visual nonverbal reasoning		✔	✔								✔	
Subtest IX: Conceptual Matching Assesses ability to categorize, associate, and reason abstractly		✔	✔			✔					✔	
Subtest X: Word Fragments Assesses ability to visually identify a familiar word with varying elements missing		✔	✔					✔				
Subtest XI: Letter Sequences Assesses ability to recall a series of letters presented visually		✔	✔		✔	✔						

Standard scores and percentiles are available for patients up to age 17-11. We would expect an adult with a high school education to score within the normal range of a 17-11 year old.

| *Developmental Test of Visual-Motor Integration (VMI)* by Keith E. Beery. Modern Curriculum Press Inc., 13900 Prospect Road, Cleveland OH 44136. | ✔ | ✔ | ✔ | | | | | ✔ | | | | |

Measures degree to which visual perception and motor behavior are integrated. The author states that this test can be used with adults even though it was developed for children. We expect our adult patients to score at the highest level which is an age equivalent of 14-6.

| *Motor-Free Visual Perception Test (MVPT)* by Ronald P. Colarusso and Donald D. Hammill. Academic Therapy Publications, 20 | | ✔ | | | | | | ✔ | | | | |

	Population			Process							
	LO	MI	HI	A	M	ORG	O	P	PR	PJ	R	S

Commercial Blvd., Novato, CA 94949.

Measures five areas of visual perception (spatial relationships, visual discrimination, figure-ground, visual closure, and visual memory) and requires no graphic response. This test was originally standardized on children. However, mean scores and standard deviations are available for adults aged 18–80 in the *Manual for Application of the Motor-Free Visual Perception Test to the Adult Population* by Mary Jane Bouska and Eugene Kwatny, P.O. Box 12246, Philadelphia, PA 19144.

Peabody Individual Achievement Test—Revised Edition by Frederick C. Markwardt Jr.
American Guidance Services, Publishers' Building, P.O. Box 99, Circle Pines, MN 55014.

General Information Subtest
Measures general encyclopedic knowledge

	LO	MI	HI	A	M	ORG	O	P	PR	PJ	R	S
General Information Subtest		✔	✔		✔							✔

Grade equivalents are available from 3.0 to 12.9. Standard scores are available up to 18-11 years of age and can be converted into percentile ranks, stanines, and normal curve equivalents. An adult with a high school education should score within the normal range for a 18-11 year old.

RIC Evaluation of Communication Problems in Right Hemisphere Dysfunction (RICE) by Martha S. Burns, Anita S. Halper, and Shelley I. Mogil
Aspen Publishers Inc., 200 Orchard Ridge Dr., Gaithersburg, MD 20878.

	Population			Process								
	LO	MI	HI	A	M	ORG	O	P	PR	PJ	R	S
Visual Scanning and Tracking Assesses ability to scan large, widely spaced and small, closely spaced letters and words		✔						✔				
Rating Scale of Pragmatic Communication Skills Measures use of nonverbal communication behaviors, conversational skills, ability to use linguistic context, and organization of discourse	✔	✔	✔						✔			
Metaphorical Language Test Assesses ability to explain the meaning of proverbs and idioms from an auditory stimulus		✔	✔								✔	
The Rivermead Behavioural Memory Test		✔	✔	✔			✔	✔				

This test is not standardized but does establish pretreatment baseline measures which can be compared to testing after treatment.

The Rivermead Behavioural Memory Test by Barbara Wilson, Janet Cockburn, Alan Baddeley.
The Thames Valley Test Company, 34/36 High Street, Titchfield, Fareham, Hants POI4 4AF, England.
Assesses everyday memory including remembering an appointment, remembering a belonging, picture recognition, immediate and delayed story recall, face recognition, remembering a short route, remembering to deliver a message, orientation and remembering a name. Two scores are available, a screening score based on a pass/fail grading of each item, and a more detailed profile score. Four parallel versions of the test are provided.

Ross Information Processing Assessment by Deborah Ross.

	Population			Process								
	LO	MI	HI	A	M	ORG	O	P	PR	PJ	R	S
Pro-Ed, 8700 Shoal Creek Blvd., Austin, TX 78758.												
Subtest I: Immediate Memory Assesses immediate recall of numbers, words, and sentences of increasing length and complexity read aloud		✔	✔	✔	✔							
Subtest II: Recent Memory Assesses recall of information related to the environment and daily activity	✔	✔	✔		✔		✔					
Subtest III: Temporal Orientation (Recent Memory) Assesses time orientation in relation to newly learned information or recent memory	✔	✔			✔		✔					
Subtest IV: Temporal Orientation (Remote Memory) Assesses remote memory of time concepts	✔	✔			✔		✔					
Subtest V: Spatial Orientation Assesses recent and remote memory of spatial (place) orientation concepts	✔	✔	✔		✔		✔					
Subtest VI: Orientation to Environment Assesses awareness and perception of the environment	✔	✔	✔		✔		✔					
Subtest VII: Recall of General Information Assesses ability to recall general information in remote memory	✔	✔			✔							
Subtest VIII: Problem Solving and Abstract Reasoning Assesses ability to problem solve and use reasoning strategies		✔	✔								✔	✔

	Population			Process								
	LO	MI	HI	A	M	ORG	O	P	PR	PJ	R	S
Subtest IX: Organization Assesses ability to name category members and recall a category name given specific category members		✔	✔			✔						✔
Subtest X: Auditory Retention and Processing Assesses ability to comprehend yes/no questions containing temporal, spatial, and comparative information		✔	✔		✔							

This test was standardized on 100 normals ranging in age from 16 to 57 and 102 patients with either closed head trauma or right hemisphere lesions between the ages of 15 and 77 years. The authors of the test found that with the exception of two items (Item 7 and 8 of subtest 8: Problem Solving and Abstract Reasoning) any difficulty with test items constitutes a deviation from normal responses. Instructions are given for scoring qualitatively using diacritical markings such as delay, perseveration, self-correction, and irrelevancy and quantitatively using a four point scale. Severity ratings are derived from the quantative score.

Ross Test of Higher Cognitive Processes by John D. Ross and Catherine M. Ross.
Academic Therapy Publications, 20 Commercial Blvd., Novato, CA 94949.

	Population			Process								
Section I: Analogies Assesses ability to identify analogous relationships between written pairs of words		✔	✔		✔						✔	

	Population			Process								
	LO	MI	HI	A	M	ORG	O	P	PR	PJ	R	S
Section II: Deductive Reasoning Assesses ability to analyze written statements to determine whether or not the conclusions follow logically			✔							✔	✔	
Section III: Missing Premises Assesses ability to identify the missing premise when given only the initial premise and the conclusion			✔							✔	✔	
Section IV: Abstract Relations Assesses ability to select from a pool of 12 words the one word that can be associated with each of four other words			✔							✔	✔	
Section V: Sequential Synthesis Assesses ability to organize ten written statements into a meaningful paragraph	✔	✔				✔					✔	
Section VI: Questioning Strategies Assesses ability to evaluate which one of three sets of written data provides the best information in determining the target item			✔							✔	✔	
Section VII: Analysis of Relevant and Irrelevant Information Assesses ability to analyze written data and determine if there is sufficient information to solve the problem and/or if irrelevant information is present			✔							✔	✔	
Section VIII: Analysis of Attributes Assesses ability to analyze and identify critical elements within a figure and determine which attributes are necessary for problem solving			✔							✔	✔	

	Population			Process								
	LO	MI	HI	A	M	ORG	O	P	PR	PJ	R	S
Percentile scores are given for grades 4–6 for each of the subtests and for the total test score. However, these norms are typically not useful because of their limited range. Performance accuracy and a qualitative analysis of the patient's approach to each task are more appropriate for the adult TBI population.												
Revised Token Test by Malcolm M. McNeil and Thomas E. Prescott. Pro-Ed, 8700 Shoal Creek Blvd., Austin, TX 78758. Assesses ability to follow more complex oral commands having minimum redundancy. Percentile ranks are available for normals and right and left hemisphere brain damaged adults 20 to 80 years of age.	✔		✔		✔							✔
Test of Problem Solving (TOPS) by Linda Zachman, Mark Barrett, Rosemary Huisingh, Carol Jorgensen. Lingui Systems, Inc., 3100 4th Ave., P.O. Box 747, East Moline, IL 61244. Assesses the five critical thinking areas of explaining inferences, determining causes of events, answering "why" questions, determining solutions, and avoiding problems. A qualitative analysis of errors is used since the test is normed on children ages 6 years to 11 years 11 months.	✔									✔	✔	
Watson-Glaser Critical Thinking Appraisal by Goodwin Watson and Edwin M. Glaser. The Psychological Corporation, P.O. Box 839954, San Antonio, TX 78283. Test 1: Inference Assesses ability to discriminate			✔							✔	✔	

	Population			Process								
	LO	MI	HI	A	M	ORG	O	P	PR	PJ	R	S

among degrees of truth or false-ness of inferences drawn from spe-cific written information

Test 2: Recognition of Assumptions
Assesses ability to identify un-stated assumptions or presupposi-tions in written statements or as-sertions ✔(HI) ✔(PJ) ✔(R)

Test 3: Deduction
Assesses ability to determine whether a conclusion follows or does not follow a written state-ment or premise ✔(HI) ✔(PJ) ✔(R)

Test 4: Interpretation
Assesses ability to determine whether or not a conclusion fol-lows beyond a reasonable doubt from the printed information ✔(HI) ✔(PJ) ✔(R)

Test 5: Evaluation of Arguments
Assesses ability to differentiate between written arguments that are strong and relevant and those that are weak or irrelevant to a particular question ✔(HI) ✔(PJ) ✔(R)

This test is useful for a select group of mildly impaired patients where critical thinking skills are es-sential for their academic or voca-tional pursuits (e.g., philosopher, journalist). The patient must have a high school degree and be able to read at the 12th grade level to per-form this test. Percentile scores are available for high school and college students.

Woodcock-Johnson Tests of Cogni-tive Ability by Richard M. Woodcock and Nancy Mather.

	Population			Process								
	LO	MI	HI	A	M	ORG	O	P	PR	PJ	R	S
DLM Teaching Resources, P.O. Box 4000, One DLM Park, Allen, TX 75002.												
Test 1: Memory for Names Measures ability to learn associations between unfamiliar auditory and visual stimuli		✔	✔		✔							
Test 2: Memory for Sentences Measures ability to repeat phrases and sentences presented auditorily via a tape player	✔	✔	✔	✔	✔							
Test 3: Visual Matching Measures ability to match two identical numbers in a row of six numbers.		✔	✔	✔				✔				
Test 4: Incomplete Words Measures ability to identify the complete word from a recorded word that has one or more phonemes missing	✔	✔	✔					✔				
Test 5: Visual Closure Measures ability to identify a drawing or picture that is distorted, has missing lines or areas, or has a superimposed pattern	✔	✔	✔					✔				
Test 6: Picture Vocabulary Measures ability to name pictures of familiar and unfamiliar objects	✔	✔	✔									✔
Test 7: Analysis-Synthesis Measures ability to analyze the components of an incomplete logic puzzle and determine the missing components		✔	✔							✔	✔	
Test 8: Visual-Auditory Learning Measures ability to associate new visual symbols with familiar		✔	✔		✔							

	Population			Process								
	LO	MI	HI	A	M	ORG	O	P	PR	PJ	R	S
words and to translate a series of symbols into verbal sentences												
Test 9: Memory for Words Measures ability to repeat in correct sequence lists of unrelated words presentedvia a tape recorder	✔	✔	✔	✔	✔							
Test 10: Cross Out Measures ability to scan and match visual information quickly		✔	✔	✔				✔				
Test 11: Sound Blending Measures ability to integrate and say whole words given parts (syllables and/or phonemes) of words via a tape recorder	✔	✔	✔					✔				
Test 12: Picture Recognition Measures ability to recognize a subset of previously presented pictures within a field of distracting pictures	✔	✔	✔		✔							
Test 13: Oral Vocabulary Measures ability to give a word similar or opposite in meaning to the word presented	✔	✔	✔									✔
Test 14: Concept Formation Measures ability to identify the rules for concepts when shown illustrations of when the rule does or does not apply		✔	✔								✔	
Test 15: Delayed Recall—Memory for Names Measures ability to recall after one to eight days the auditory-visual associations presented in Test 1		✔	✔		✔							
Test 16: Delayed Recall—Visual-Auditory Learning Measures ability to recall after one		✔	✔		✔							

	Population			Process								
	LO	MI	HI	A	M	ORG	O	P	PR	PJ	R	S
to eight days the symbols presented in Test 8												
Test 17: Numbers Reversed Measures ability to say in reverse order a series of numbers presented via a tape recorder	✔	✔	✔	✔	✔							
Test 18: Sound Patterns Measures ability to indicate whether pairs of complex sound patterns presented via a tape recorder are the same or different	✔	✔	✔					✔				
Test 19: Spatial Relations Measures ability to identify from a series of shapes, the component parts required to make a given whole shape		✔	✔					✔			✔	
Test 20: Listening Comprehension Measures ability to listen to a tape-recorded sentence or paragraph and supply the single word missing at the end of it	✔	✔	✔		✔						✔	
Test 21: Verbal Analogies Measures ability to complete phrases with words that indicate appropriate analogies	✔	✔	✔				✔				✔	

Rank order, standard scores, and percentile ranks are available for ages 2 to 90+ and grades kindergarten through 16.9. With older patients it is more useful to use the age norms while for younger patients who may be returning to school, it is preferable to use the grade norms.

The Adolescent Word Test by Linda Zachman, Mark Barrett, Rosemary Huisingh, Jane Orman and Carolyn Bladgen.
LinguiSystems, 3100 4th Avenue,

	Population			Process								
	LO	MI	HI	A	M	ORG	O	P	PR	PJ	R	S

P.O. Box 747, East Moline, IL 61244.

Task A: Brand Names
Assesses ability to indicate why the name of a product or company is appropriate

	LO	MI	HI	A	M	ORG	O	P	PR	PJ	R	S
Task A: Brand Names		✔	✔								✔	

Task B: Synonyms
Assesses ability to provide a synonym for a given word presented in a sentence

	LO	MI	HI	A	M	ORG	O	P	PR	PJ	R	S
Task B: Synonyms		✔	✔									✔

Task C: Signs of the Times
Assesses ability to explain the meaning of a functional sign or message and provide the reason for its importance

	LO	MI	HI	A	M	ORG	O	P	PR	PJ	R	S
Task C: Signs of the Times		✔	✔								✔	

Task D: Definitions
Assesses ability to define a given word

	LO	MI	HI	A	M	ORG	O	P	PR	PJ	R	S
Task D: Definitions		✔	✔									✔

Standard scores and percentile ranks are available for ages 12-0 through 17-11. An individual over this age would be expected to score in the normal range for 17-11 year olds.

The Word Test by Carol Jorgensen, Mark Barrett, Rosemary Huisingh, and Linda Zachman.
LinguiSystems, 3100 4th Avenue, P.O. Box 747, East Moline, IL 61244.

Task A: Associations
Assesses ability to identify the one word from a group that does not belong

	LO	MI	HI	A	M	ORG	O	P	PR	PJ	R	S
Task A: Associations	✔	✔			✔							✔

Task B: Synonyms
Assesses ability to provide a synonym for a given word

	LO	MI	HI	A	M	ORG	O	P	PR	PJ	R	S
Task B: Synonyms	✔	✔										✔

| | Population | | | Process | | | | | | | | |
	LO	MI	HI	A	M	ORG	O	P	PR	PJ	R	S
Task C: Semantic Absurdities Assesses ability to explain or correct sentences that are semantically absurd	✔	✔									✔	
Task D: Antonyms Assesses ability to provide an antonym for a given word	✔	✔										✔
Task E: Definitions Assesses ability to give meanings of words	✔	✔										✔
Task F: Multiple Definitions Assesses ability to give two meanings of a word	✔	✔									✔	✔

A qualitative analysis of errors is used since the test is normed on children ages 7 years through 11 years 11 months.

Language-Related Academic Tests

Adult Basic Learning Examination (ABLE): Levels I, II, III by Bjorn Karlsen and Eric F. Gardner. The Psychological Corporation, 555 Academic Court, San Antonio, TX 78204-2498.

Level 1 measures vocabulary, reading comprehension, spelling, number operations, and arithmetic problem solving. Levels 2 and 3 measure these areas as well as applied grammar, capitalization, and punctuation. This test was designed specifically for the adult population. Level I is appropriate for adults with one to four years of education, Level II for five to eight years of education, and Level III for those who have had at least eight years of schooling. Scaled scores, percentile ranks, stanines, and grade equivalents are provided.

Gates-MacGinitie Reading Survey Tests: Levels 4, 5/6, 7/9, 10/12 (3rd edition) by Walter H. MacGinitie and Ruth K. MacGinitie. The Riverside Publishing Co., 8420 Bryn Mawr Ave., Chicago, IL 60631.

Measures reading vocabulary and comprehension. Norms are provided for grades 4 through 12 with extended scaled scores, percentile ranks, stanines, and grade equivalents given.

Iowa Silent Reading Tests: Levels 1, 2, 3 edited by Roger Farr. The Psychological Corporation, 555 Academic Court, San Antonio, TX 78204.

Level 1, appropriate for grades 6–9, assesses vocabulary, reading comprehension, and directed reading. Level 2, appropriate for grades 9–14, assesses these areas in addition to reading efficiency. Level 3, appropriate for academically accelerated high school and college students, assesses vocabulary, reading comprehension, and reading efficiency. Percentile ranks, stanine scores, and standard scores are available for grades 6 through 12 and college students.

Keymath Revised: A Diagnostic Inventory of Essential Mathematics by Austin J. Connolly. American Guidance Service, Publishers' Building, P.O. Box 99, Circle Pines, MN 55014-.

Measures basic mathematical concepts (numeration, rational numbers, and geometry), arithmetic operations (addition, subtraction, multiplication, division, and mental computations), and functional applications (measurement, time and money, estimation, interpreting data, and problem solving. Standard scores, grade and age equivalents, percentile ranks, and stanines are available for kindergarten through grade 9 and ages 5.0–15.11.

Metropolitan Achievement Tests, Sixth Edition (MAT 6) Survey Battery: Elementary, Intermediate, Advanced 1 and 2 by George A. Prescott, Irving H. Balow, Thomas P. Hogan, and Roger C. Farr. The Psychological Corporation, 555 Academic Court, San Antonio, TX 78204-2498.

Assesses achievement in the areas of reading (vocabulary, word recognition, and reading comprehension), mathematics (concepts, problem solving, and computation), language, social studies, and science. Norms given include scaled scores, percentile ranks, stanines, and grade equivalents. The Elementary level is appropriate for grades 3.5–4.9; the Intermediate level for grades 5.0–6.9; Advanced 1 for grades 7.0–9.9; and Advanced 2 for grades 10.0–12.9.

Peabody Individual Achievement Test—Revised (PIAT-R) by Frederick C. Markwardt, Jr. American Guidance Services, Publishers' Building, P.O. Box 99, Circle Pines, MN 55014.

Measures general information, reading recognition, reading comprehension, mathematics, spelling, and written expression. Age and grade-based standard scores, age and grade equivalents, percentile ranks, and stanines are provided for ages 5–18.11 and grades K–12.

Quick-Score Achievement Test by Donald D. Hammill, Jerome J. Ammer, Mary E. Cronin, Linda H. Mandlebaum, and Sally S. Quinby.
Pro-Ed, 8700 Shoal Creek Blvd., Austin, TX 78758.

Assesses proficiency in reading, writing, arithmetic, and factual information related to science, social studies, health, and language arts. Percentiles and standard scores are provided for ages 7-0 to 17-11.

Stanford Achievement Test Series, Eighth Edition: Intermediate 1, 2, 3, Advanced 1, 2, Task 1, 2, 3 by Eric F. Gardner, Herbert C. Rudman, Bjorn Karlsen, Jack C. Merwin, Richard Madden, Cathy S. Collins, and Robert Callis.
The Psychological Corporation, 555 Academic Court, San Antonio, TX 78204.

Assesses reading vocabulary and comprehension, language, study skills, spelling, listening, number concepts, computations, arithmetic applications, science, and social science. Scaled scores, percentile ranks, stanines, and grade equivalents are provided for grades 4–12.9.

Tests of Achievement and Proficiency by Dale P. Scannell, Oscar M. Haugh, Alvin H. Schild, and Gilbert Ulmer.
The Riverside Publishing Co., 8420 Bryn Mawr Ave., Chicago, IL 60631.

Assesses reading comprehension, mathematics, written expression (e.g., spelling, punctuation, grammar) using sources of information, social studies, science, listening, and essay writing. Standard scores, stanines, percentile ranks, and grade equivalents are available for grades 9–12.

Test of Written Language—2 (TOWL-2) by Donald D. Hammill and Stephen C. Larsen.
Pro-Ed, 8700 Shoal Creek Blvd., Austin, TX 78758.

Assesses spontaneous written output as well as vocabulary, style and spelling, logical sentences, and combining sentences. Percentile and standard scores are provided for ages 7.0–17.11.

Woodcock-Johnson Tests of Achievement by Richard W. Woodcock and Nancy Mather.
DLM Teaching Resources, One DLM Park, Allen, TX 75002.

Assesses reading (letter-word identification, passage comprehension, word attack, and reading vocabulary), mathematics (calculation, applied problems, and quantitative concepts), written language (dictation, writing samples, proofing, writing fluency, punctuation and capitalization, spelling, usage, handwriting), and knowledge (science, social studies, and humanities). Norms are available for ages 2 to 90+ and grades kindergarten through grade 16.9.

Woodcock Reading Mastery Tests—Revised by Richard W. Woodcock.
American Guidance Service, Publishers' Building, P.O. Box 99, Circle Pines, MN 55014.

Measures word identification, word attack, word comprehension (antonyms, synonyms, analogies), and passage comprehension. Percentile ranks, standard scores, age equivalents, and grade equivalents are available for ages 5–75+ and grades kindergarten through 16.9.

Chapter 5

Treatment of Communication Problems

Leora R. Cherney, Anita S. Halper, and Trudy K. Miller

The treatment of cognitive-linguistic deficits that result in communicative and executive problems is presented in this chapter. Our approach is process-specific[1] and directed toward those processes discussed in previous chapters. The information provided is intended as a treatment guide to aid the speech-language pathologist in choosing appropriate goals, carrying out a treatment plan, and documenting progress.

While each process is addressed separately, the clinician typically works on more than one process at a time. The goals and procedures within each process are presented in a hierarchical format. However, this order may need to be modified according to the patient's strengths and weaknesses and unique needs and interests.

A means of measuring the patient's performance accompanies each procedure. These measurements can be incorporated into written goals. For example, the goal of increasing awareness of and responsiveness to auditory stimulation, specifically music, can be measured by the number and type of responses in a designated time period. The goal then could be written as: patient will localize to music source two to three times in a 15 minute time period.

It is important that the speech-language pathologist differentiate between testing and teaching the patient. Testing, which involves determining the patient's level of performance on a given task, is useful for establishing baseline performance. Teaching includes providing the patient with structure, cues, and strategies so that maximum performance on a given task can be achieved. For example, reading a story and then asking questions related to it is testing. However, if the patient is first directed to listen for specific ideas (e.g., the who, what, when, and where of the story) the task becomes a teaching one because the patient is provided with a listening strategy. Therefore, it is useful during teaching to measure not only the patient's accuracy of performance but also the type and number of cues provided. A change or decrease in the cues given by the clinician or a shift from clinician-generated to patient-generated cues reflects progress.

Perhaps the most difficult aspect of treatment is the generalization of the patient's performance to everyday situations outside the treatment session. The involvement of family/caregivers and all staff is essential for carry-over of skills to the natural environment.[2] A setting that allows for education of and ongoing communication among team members, families, patients, and other staff will facilitate this carry-over of skills.

Family involvement should begin early in treatment and continue throughout the rehabilitation process regardless of the level of the patient. For example, family and staff should be involved in providing sensory stimulation to the patient with reduced awareness and responsiveness (a discussion of sensory stimulation follows in this chapter). At the other end of the severity continuum, family and staff can encourage the patient with mild deficits to generalize problem-solving strategies learned in treatment to situations encountered at home or on the nursing unit. Chapter 6 discusses the role of the family in the rehabilitation of the person with traumatic brain injury.

In addition to individual treatment, group treatment is an effective means of rehabilitation for this population.[1] Two interdisciplinary groups that include staff from physical, occupational, and recreational therapies as well as speech-language pathology have been developed at the Rehabilitation Institute of Chicago. The Life Skills Group is designed to meet the needs of the moderately impaired patient, while the Independent Living Skills Group is designed to facilitate re-entry of the mildly impaired patient into the community. Both groups focus on fostering appropriate use of pragmatic skills and interaction between patients. The groups plan and execute activities that are relevant to everyday life and receive feedback on their performance.

There are a variety of published materials and computer programs which can be used directly or adapted for treating a specific cognitive-linguistic process. Appendix 5-A is an annotated list of materials and Appendix 5-B is an annotated list of software programs. Both appendices include the processes for which the treatment materials and computer programs might be used. When selecting treatment activities, it is important to recognize that completion of a given task may require more than one process. Therefore, the clinician should analyze each task to determine which cognitive-linguistic processes are involved and modify the activity to emphasize the targeted process. Computerized activities are a useful adjunct to treatment for some patients but should not be used to the exclusion of more functional activities.

SENSORY STIMULATION

Sensory stimulation may be defined as the systematic application of multimodality stimuli to increase the patient's alertness/arousal and responsiveness to the environment and to prevent sensory deprivation. This program is appropriate for patients who are emerging from a nonresponsive state and whose responses to their environment are minimal.[3] These are the patients who were classified as Level 1, with reduced alertness/arousal and responsiveness, in Chapter 4. In the early stages of recovery, sensory stimulation procedures require no active participation on the part of the patient. Gradually, the procedures require that the patient participate more actively and make more purposeful responses. The goals and procedures included early in the hierarchy of treatment for attention, orientation, and perception also may be appropriate for patients in a sensory stimulation program.

The role of the speech-language pathologist is twofold. The first role is to provide daily brief periods of sensory stimulation to facilitate changes in responsiveness such as increased consistency and specificity of response and/or decreased latency of response. The second role is to provide training to family and/or caregivers who then can carry out many of these activities independently.

Smith and Ylvisaker[3] have presented a rationale for beginning with vestibular, tactile, olfactory, and gustatory stimulation before proceeding to auditory and visual stimulation. These sensory systems are phylogenetically older and are represented subcortically as compared to the auditory and visual systems, which are cortically represented. Further, these subcortical systems may suffer less primary damage.[4]

Depending on the individual patient, it may be best to first present single modality stimulation and later move to multimodality stimulation. When more than one system is stimulated simultaneously, the stimuli should be meaningfully related. For example, simultaneously ringing a bell while smelling banana extract does not allow the patient to integrate the stimuli meaningfully. Simultaneously smelling and tasting the banana extract, or seeing and ringing the bell is preferable.

The type, rate, intensity, and duration of the stimuli should be carefully controlled to facilitate the best response from the patient. Although noxious stimuli may be used during the evaluation to assess the patient's responsiveness, we avoid using noxious stimuli for treatment because it may have an adverse effect on the patient. It is also important for the speech-language pathologist to explore with the family those sensory stimuli that the patient responded to favorably premorbidly. Presentation of stimuli should be appropriate to the patient's response rate. It is important to allow adequate time for the patient to respond because speed of processing is reduced. Sensory stimulation should not be continuous; the type, intensity, and duration of the stimuli should be varied to avoid habituation of the response.[3] In addition, the sensory stimulation session should be brief (15 to 20 minutes) and occur several times a day.

Patient responses can be categorized according to the seven point scale described in Chapter 4. These are as follows: consistent related localized response; consistent unrelated localized response; inconsistent related localized response; inconsistent unrelated localized response; consistent generalized response; inconsistent generalized response; and no response. In addition, the types of responses elicited from an individual patient should be noted. These may include changes in physiological status (e.g., change in skin color or respiratory rate), body and facial movements, oral-motor responses, and vocalizations.

The speech-language pathologist has an important role as a member of the interdisciplinary sensory stimulation team. At the Rehabilitation Institute of Chicago, the speech-language pathologist, the physical and occupational therapists, and the neuropsychologist each administer sensory stimulation during brief individual sessions at different times of day. The patient's responses are recorded on the same data form (Exhibit 5-1) regardless of who is administering the stimulation. Therefore, the form includes some terms that are not specific to speech-language pathology. The team meets periodically to review the patient's progress and revise the program accordingly.

During this initial phase of treatment, the family/significant others observe the speech-language pathologist administering sensory stimulation. The family members learn the appropriate techniques for providing sensory stimulation through this observation together with practice. They are also taught how to identify and record the type, consistency, and latency of response. Exhibit 5-2 shows the simplified recording form used by family members. Note that taste has been omitted to prevent oral intake and the possibility of aspiration. The speech-language pathologist reviews the data collected by family members periodically with the team.

Every patient involved in a sensory stimulation program is supplied with a stimulation kit. The use of a common set of stimuli facilitates consistency among the different disciplines in stimulus presentation. The sensory stimulation kit includes the following:

- food extracts
- Q-tips
- scrubbing sponge with both a smooth and rough surface
- comb and brush
- cotton balls
- feathers
- washcloth
- metal spoon
- pins
- tongue depressors
- vibrator
- balloons
- brightly colored objects (e.g., balls, blocks, rings)
- flashlight
- laryngeal mirror

- noisemakers (e.g., bell, maraca, squeak toy)
- recording forms

These items form a core of stimuli that are useful for all patients. However, additional items are added based on the individual patient's premorbid personal preferences (e.g., cologne, soap, coffee).

Early involvement of the speech-language pathologist in the sensory stimulation program is necessary to identify changes in the patient's responsiveness, particularly to auditory, visual, and oral-motor stimuli. These changes may indicate that the patient is ready for a more active cognitive-linguistic treatment program. However, if a patient does not demonstrate changes in responsiveness after an intensive period of sensory stimulation, then daily treatment by the speech-language pathologist is discontinued. We feel that three to four weeks is usually sufficient to make this determination. The family and other caregivers are then instructed to continue sensory stimulation several times a day. The speech-language pathologist observes at least weekly the family members providing sensory stimulation to ensure appropriate administration and recording. The physical and occupational therapists, who continue to see the patient daily for activities such as positioning and range of motion, may also provide sensory stimulation. The speech-language pathologist reviews the patient response forms and sees the patient weekly to identify any changes in status.

Sensory stimulation activities that focus primarily on the auditory, visual, and oral-motor areas are described in the following procedures. These are emphasized because of their importance to communication and feeding. There are other types of sensory stimulation that may be appropriate for a particular patient (e.g., vestibular). However, occupational and physical therapists often are better trained to provide such stimulation.

Goal	Procedure	Measurement	Comments
1. Increase awareness of and responsiveness to sensory stimulation.			
a. Tactile	Provide tactile stimulation to the face using: • Light touch (e.g., feather, cotton balls) • Deep touch/massage • Vibration (e.g., vibrator) • Textures (e.g., scrubbing sponges/soft sponge) • Thermal input (e.g., hot and cold washcloths)	Number and type of responses in a designated time period.	
	Provide tactile stimulation to the lips, tongue, gums, and cheeks via: • Light touch with a tongue depressor or toothbrush • Deep touch/massage with a tongue depressor or spoon • Tapping the structures with a tongue depressor or spoon • Thermal input with a laryngeal mirror or metal spoon dipped in ice or warm water.	Same as above.	Slow, even and rhythmical stimulation is appropriate for hypertonic muscles to inhibit hypertonicity; quick, uneven and intermittent stimulation is appropriate for hypotonic muscles to facilitate increased tone.[5]
b. Olfactory	Provide pleasant olfactory stimuli such as: • Personal smells (e.g., cologne, hairspray, shampoo) • Food extracts (e.g., banana, vanilla, peppermint) • Food aromas (e.g., popcorn, oranges, coffee).	Number and type of responses in a designated time period.	
c. Gustatory	Provide pleasant gustatory stimuli to the lips, gums, cheeks, and tongue using Q-tips dipped in fruit juices, gravies, soups, and sauces.	Number and type of responses in a designated time period.	Caution should be taken with patients who have feeding problems.
d. Auditory	Present a variety of noises such as bells, squeak toys, drums, maracas,	Number and type of responses in a	

Goal	Procedure	Measurement	Comments
	a ticking clock, and hand clapping.	designated time period.	
	Present music and: • Alternate loudness levels • Alternate side to which music is presented • Alternate type of music presented (e.g., rock, classical).	Same as above.	Music should be played intermittently so that the patient also has periods of silence.
	Call the patient's name periodically.	Same as above.	
	Present a simple monologue about the patient using either live voices or tapes of family members.	Same as above.	
e. Visual	Present light by • Turning room lights on and off • Shining penlight into or across patient's eyes • Opening and closing shades.	Number and type of responses in a designated time period.	
2. Establish eye contact with speaker.	Manipulate patient's head and use verbal cues with exaggerated vocal inflection and gestures to establish eye contact with the clinician.	Number of times head must be manipulated and/or type and number of cues required to establish eye contact in a designated time period.	Caution needs to be taken with the agitated patient.
3. Focus visual gaze to treatment materials.	Hold large, bright, contrasting colored objects in patient's visual field. Cue as above.	Number of times eye gaze is focused to object, and/or type and number of cues required to establish eye gaze in a designated time period.	
	Hold family pictures and/or brightly colored pictures in patient's visual field. Use cues as above.	Same as above.	

Exhibit 5-1 Sensory Stimulation Response Form: Interdisciplinary Team

Key to Responses:
6—Consistent, related localized
5—Consistent, unrelated localized
4—Inconsistent, related localized
3—Inconsistent, unrelated localized
2—Consistent generalized
1—Inconsistent generalized
0—No response

	Date					
	Time					
	Clinician					
	Department					
TACTILE	Surface Pain					
	Deep Pain					
	Light Touch					
	Deep Touch/Massage					
	Vibration					
	Textures					
	Thermal					
	Comments:					
KINES/VESTIB	Passive movement					
	Assistive movement					
	Rolling					
	Supine to sitting					
	Rocking					
	Comments:					
OLF	Personal odors					
	Food odors					
	Comments:					
GUST	Taste					
	Comments:					
AUDITORY	Noises					
	Music					
	Patient's name					
	Simple conversation					
	Comments:					
VISUAL	Protective blink					
	Light					
	Eye contact					
	Focus on objects/pictures					
	Tracking					
	Comments:					

Exhibit 5-2 Sensory Stimulation Response Form: Family

Patient _____ Date _____

Stimulation	*Type, Consistency and Timeliness of Response*
Day _____ Touch Movement Smell Hearing Vision	
Day _____ Touch Movement Smell Hearing Vision	
Day _____ Touch Movement Smell Hearing Vision	
Day _____ Touch Movement Smell Hearing Vision	
Day _____ Touch Movement Smell Hearing Vision	

ATTENTION

Attention is an important element in the treatment of all patients with traumatic brain injury. Attentional deficits at all levels need to be addressed. For example, both the patient emerging from coma with reduced alertness/arousal and nonresponsiveness and the patient having difficulty with divided attention for such tasks as listening to a lecture and taking notes simultaneously require treatment. In the early stages, the major goal of treatment is to improve focused and sustained attention. Initially, accuracy is not a useful measure of the patient's success, so it is important to use easy, nonfrustrating tasks. Once a level of sustained attention sufficient for task completion is achieved, task complexity can be increased gradually. Accuracy then becomes a relevant measure of the patient's performance. A qualitative analysis of errors may provide additional information about the patient's performance and progress. For example, decreased accuracy at the beginning of a task may indicate difficulty establishing a new set and may reflect problems in shifting attention. In contrast, decreased accuracy at the end of a task may indicate problems with sustained attention.[2]

Goal	Procedure	Measurement	Comments
1. Increase sustained attention.			
a. Maintain eye contact with speaker.	Present conversation related to the patient and have patient maintain eye contact: • Use tactile, gestural and/or verbal cues with exaggerated vocal inflection as needed • Decrease cues gradually and increase the number of speakers.	Length of time patient maintains eye contact and type and number of cues required to maintain eye contact for the designated time period.	
b. Maintain visual attention to pictures.	Present family pictures or other familiar pictures and have patient maintain eye gaze. Use above cues and gradually decrease.	Length of time patient maintains eye gaze and type and number of cues required to maintain eye gaze.	
c. Maintain visual attention to moving targets.	Move brightly colored and contrasting objects, a mirror, flashlight, or pictures across the patient's visual field and have patient follow visually. Use above cues and gradually decrease.	Length of time patient maintains gaze on moving target and type and number of cues required to maintain eye gaze.	Start with moving targets horizontally or vertically depending on which movements are easier for the patient.
d. Maintain attention to a task.	Present the following matching tasks and have patient perform: • matching colors	Length of time patient attends to task and/or type and	Once a level of sustained attention sufficient for task

Goal	Procedure	Measurement	Comments
	• matching geometric forms • matching letters and numbers • matching identical objects and pictures • matching similar objects and pictures. Use above cues as necessary to reestablish patient's attention to task.	number of cues required to regain patient's attention in a designated time period.	completion is attained, a measure of accuracy can be introduced. The goal is to retain the same level of sustained attention while increasing accuracy of performance.
	Present the following scanning tasks and have patient perform: • scanning of colors and shapes • scanning of letters and numbers • scanning of pictures and words • simple trailmaking exercises (see Exhibit 5-3). Use above cues as necessary to reestablish patient's attention to task.	Same as above.	These tasks and the matching tasks above are also appropriate for treatment of perceptual problems.
	Present playing cards one at a time and have patient add the numbers on each card to the previous sum (see Exhibit 5-4).	Same as above.	If the task requirements are periodically changed from addition to subtraction and back again, this then becomes an activity for improving ability to shift attention (see Exhibit 5-4).
2. Improve selective attention.	Introduce competing visual and/or auditory stimuli in the following ways and have patient perform the above matching and scanning tasks: • increase number of items in the visual field • play audio tapes of environmental noises (e.g., cafeteria noise, traffic, playground sounds) • turn on the radio/television in the background	Percent correct, length of attention to task, and type and number of cues required to regain attention in a designated time period.	

Goal	Procedure	Measurement	Comments
	• open door to the hall • take patient outside the treatment room into the lobby. Increase gradually the amount of distraction.		
	Present an auditory or visual list and have patient identify the target letter/number/word every time it occurs: • Use verbal and/or gestural cues and gradually decrease • Increase gradually the length of the list and the similarity between the target and the foil (orthographic, semantic, syntactic, phonetic) (see Exhibit 5-5). • Increase gradually the rate of auditorally presented material.	Percent correct and type and number of cues required to redirect attention.	
	Present an auditory or visual story and have patient identify the target word every time it occurs (see Exhibit 5-6): • Use above cues and gradually decrease • Increase length and complexity of story.	Percent correct and type and number of cues required to redirect attention.	
3. Improve ability to shift attentional set.			
a. Shift attention from task to task.	Choose two tasks that are successful for the patient and have patient alternately perform each task. Use verbal and/or gestural cues and gradually decrease.	Number of appropriate shifts in a designated time period, length of time required to change attentional set, and/or type and number of cues required to make a shift.	For some patients shifting from an auditory to visual task or vice versa may be easier than shifting to a task within the same modality.
b. Shift attention from task to nontask to task.	Present a task that is successful for the patient, introduce an interrupting activity (e.g., answering phone, conversation), and have patient return to the original task. Use	Number of appropriate shifts in a designated time period, length of time required to change	Gradually modify the length of the interrupting activity. For some patients, shorter

Goal	Procedure	Measurement	Comments
	above cues and gradually decrease.	attentional set, and/or type and number of cues required to make a shift.	interruptions are more difficult, while longer interruptions are more difficult for others.
c. Shift attention within a task.	Present a scanning task that is easy for the patient and have patient perform it while periodically changing the task requirement or the response requirement (see Exhibit 5-7).	Percent of appropriate shifts and length of time required to change attentional set.	
4. Improve ability to attend to two tasks simultaneously.	Present a task that is successful for the patient. Introduce another activity (e.g., conversation, talking, on the telephone, listening to the radio): • Have patient continue to complete the original task while simultaneously performing the new task • Increase gradually complexity and abstractness of the new task.	Length of time patient attends to both activities simultaneously, type and number of cues required to maintain divided attention, and percent correct.	
5. Increase sustained attention (concentration) to task over a longer period of time.	Present any level of treatment activities and have patient perform. Use verbal and gestural cues to redirect patient's attention.	Length of time from initiation of task to time patient stops attending and type and number of cues required to redirect patient throughout treatment session/task.	

Exhibit 5-3 Example of Trailmaking Exercise

Directions: Draw a line to connect the letters in alphabetical order.

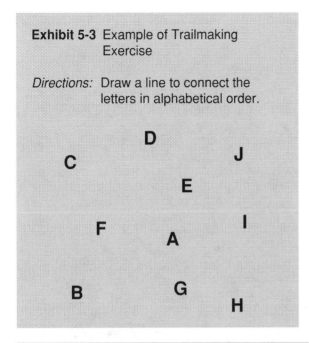

Exhibit 5-4 Example of Playing Card Activity

Directions: Keep adding these cards together until I tell you to start subtracting them.

Task Requirement	Visual Stimulus (Card)	Expected Response
Addition	3 + 7	10
	+ 5	15
	+ 2	17
Subtraction	− 9	8
	− 2	6
	− 5	1
Addition	+ 4	5

Exhibit 5-5 Selecting Target Word from List

Example of Orthographic Similarities

fish: dish, fist, tish, fisk, wish, bish, fash, fast

Example of Semantic Similarities

pretty: beautiful, cute, lovely, nice, attractive, striking

Example of Phonetic Similarities

cat: hat, mat, sat, pat, rat, gat, gnat, cap, cad

Example of Syntactic Similarities

jump: jumped, jumping, jumps

Example of an Exercise for Selecting Target Word

Directions: Circle the word "jump" every time you see it (raise your hand every time you hear the word "jump").

jump champ leap jumping hop lamp jump lump jam
jumps dump pump clump clamp jump climb jumped
camp skip rump jump bump hump jim chimp jump

Exhibit 5-6 Identifying Target Word from a Story

Directions: Circle the word "fishing" every time you see it (raise your hand every time you hear the word "fishing").

It was a hot summer day when my father came into the room and announced that we were going fishing. I had never been fishing so I was quite excited about it. There were many things we needed for the fishing trip. First, we had to buy rods, reels, and fish bait. Then my father remembered we needed a fishing license. While he picked up the license my mother packed a picnic basket. Finally we were on our way.

Exhibit 5-7 Example of Shifting Attention Task

Directions: Circle the letter "A" until I tell you to do something else.

N	P	A	E	C	R	A	G	T	A
A	S	F	D	Q	G	R	C	A	B
D	V	J	A	A	A	O	I	Z	E
U	Y	S	P	Z	X	M	A	N	O

Changing the Task Requirements:

- Circle another letter
- Circle more than one letter at a time
- Circle all vowels or all consonants
- Circle a letter only when it follows or precedes another given letter

Changing the Response Requirements:

- Underline the target
- Cross out the target

ORIENTATION

A continuum of orientation problems is present in the traumatic brain injured patient. At one end is the patient who is disoriented to person, place, situation, and time primarily as a result of attentional and perceptual problems. In this case, the goal of treatment is to increase the patient's awareness of the environment and help develop more appropriate perceptions of the real world. At the other end of the continuum is the patient who is disoriented to time and place primarily because of an underlying memory deficit. Treatment would then focus on the development of compensatory strategies for the memory problem.

Orientation to person typically improves first, followed by orientation to place and circumstances. Further, the extent to which environmental and situational cues are present help determine which aspects of orientation will improve first.[1] For example, the nurse who is constantly around the patient may be recognized before the speech-language pathologist. Recognizing that this person is a nurse may lead to the realization of being in a hospital before remembering the circumstances leading to hospitalization. Orientation to time improves last because of the dynamic nature of time; the information changes constantly.[1]

It is often helpful to consider a hierarchy of goals when developing treatment activities. Passive orientation to time and place should be treated before active orientation.[6] For example, patients will need to learn where they are in their environment (passive) before they can learn to find their way around the environment (active). Similarly, patients will need to know how to tell time (passive) before they can monitor the passage of time (active).

Goal	Procedure	Measurement	Comments
1. Establish orientation to person.			
a. Establish orientation to self.	Review personal information such as name, age, and occupation and have patient repeat facts: • Immediately • After a brief delay • After intervening orientation facts • After intervening tasks. Use visual cues including photographs and a mirror as needed to make stimuli more meaningful.	Percent correct, number of stimulus repetitions, and/or type and number of cues required to obtain accurate response.	
b. Establish orientation to significant persons.	Review names, relationships, and any other pertinent information and have patient repeat: • Immediately • After a brief delay • After intervening orientation facts • After intervening tasks. Cue with photographs, audio/video recordings, and by identifying distinctive characteristics of the specific person.	Percent correct, number of stimulus repetitions, and/or type and number of cues required to obtain accurate response.	

Goal	Procedure	Measurement	Comments
c. Establish orientation to staff.	Review name, role, and function of staff member and have patient: • Identify whether staff member is familiar or unfamiliar (e.g., Have you seen me before?) • Identify general role (e.g., therapist versus maintenance staff) • Identify specific role (e.g., speech-language pathologist versus nurse) • Describe function • Name staff person. Have patient respond: • Immediately • After a brief delay • After intervening orientation facts • After intervening tasks. Cue with pictures and by identifying distinctive characteristics of each staff member. Increase gradually number of staff reviewed.	Percent correct, number of stimulus repetitions, and/or type and number of cues required to obtain accurate response.	
2. Establish passive orientation to place.	Present objects typical to the environment and have patient identify the general location in which they belong (see Exhibit 5-8).	Percent correct, number of stimulus repetitions, and/or number and type of cues required to obtain accurate response.	
	Present the above objects and have patient identify the specific location in which they can be found (see Exhibit 5-8).	Same as above.	
	Review place orientation facts such as name of facility, address, and location of specific treatment areas and have patient repeat facts: • Immediately • After a brief delay • After intervening orientation facts • After intervening tasks.	Same as above.	

Goal	Procedure	Measurement	Comments
	Cue with objects in the environment.		
3. Establish orientation to situation.	Review the circumstances of the patient's accident and subsequent problems and have the patient repeat facts: • Immediately • After a brief delay • After intervening orientation facts • After intervening tasks. Cue with "wh" questions.	Percent correct, number of stimulus repetitions, and/or number of cues required to obtain accurate response.	
4. Establish passive orientation to time.	Present temporal cues (e.g., calendars, daily schedules, clocks) and environmental cues (e.g., dark versus light, snow versus green grass) and have patient tell: • day versus night • morning versus afternoon • time • day of the week • month • day of the month • year • season Decrease gradually the number of cues provided.	Percent correct, type and number of cues required, and/or number of self-generated versus clinician generated cues.	
5. Establish active orientation to place.	Accompany patient to a specific destination while verbally identifying environmental cues along the way. Review the route verbally and have patient follow the route.	Type and number of cues required.	Cues may be a natural part of the environment or may be specially placed by the clinician for a specific patient (e.g., sign with patient's name indicating the direction to his/her room).
	Ask patient to go from one location to another: • Cue as necessary • Gradually increase the length and complexity of the route.	Accuracy of route, number of self-generated versus clinician-generated cues, and/or time	

Goal	Procedure	Measurement	Comments
		necessary to find destination.	
6. Establish schematic representation of place.	Present maps and floor plans and have patient answer questions about the diagram (see Exhibit 5-9). Move from simple diagrams of the patient's personal environment to more complicated diagrams of remote locations.	Percent correct.	This task may require visual perceptual and problem solving skills.
7. Establish active orientation to time.	Have patient indicate when a given time period has ended (e.g., "Tell me when five minutes has ended") or estimate the amount of time that has elapsed since the beginning of an activity (e.g., "How long have we been working on this activity?")	Time variance between actual time period and the patient's estimate.	
	Have patient estimate the time it takes to perform routine activities: • Use verbal cues such as the sequence of steps involved in completing the activity • Move from simple (e.g., brushing teeth) to complex activities (e.g., Christmas shopping).	Time variance between clinician's and patient's estimates and/or number of cues required.	

Exhibit 5-8 Example of Objects and Their Location

Object	General Location	Specific Location
Stethoscope	Hospital	Doctor's office/around doctor's or nurse's neck
White coats	Hospital	On hospital staff
Parallel bars	Hospital	Physical Therapy
Nursing station	Hospital	Patient Floors
Stove	Home	Kitchen
Sofa	Home	Living Room/Family Room
Flowers	Outside	Ground/Garden
Organ	Church/Synagogue	Altar/Choir Loft
Hammer	Home/Workplace	Tool Box/Workbench/Basement
Typewriter	Home/Workplace	Desk/Office

Exhibit 5-9 Activities for Maps and Floor Plans

Map
  1. Identify the location of specific cities, states, rivers, highways, etc.
  2. Explain the relationship of one place to another (e.g., south, north, east, west).
  3. Follow a given route between two points.
  4. Explain how to get from one point to another.
  5. Give alternate routes to get from one point to another.
  6. Estimate the distance between two points.

Floor Plan
  1. Identify the location of specific rooms.
  2. Identify the number of specific bedrooms, doorways, closets, floors, etc.
  3. Explain the relationship of one room to another (above, below, right, left).
  4. Follow the route from one room to another.
  5. Explain how to get from one room to another.
  6. Compare the sizes of specific rooms.

PERCEPTION

The visual and auditory perceptual deficits of the traumatic brain injured patient may be due to specific perceptual deficits such as visuospatial or auditory closure problems or may result from difficulty with other processes such as attention, organization, problem solving, and semantics.[7] This section will focus on the rehabilitation of perceptual problems per se. It does not include treatment for visual-motor deficits because in many settings, including our own, these problems are treated by the occupational therapist. Many of the matching, scanning, trail-making, and vigilance exercises described for treatment of attention are also useful in the area of perception.

Goal	Procedure	Measurement	Comments
1. Develop recognition of environmental sounds.	Present environmental noises (e.g., telephone ringing, familiar voices, television) and have patient identify the noises either by pointing to a picture or naming them.	Percent correct.	
2. Improve auditory perceptual skills.			
a. Develop auditory discrimination.	Present pairs of words and have patient identify whether the words are the same or different. Increase gradually the similarity between the words, decrease the familiarity of the words, and increase length.	Percent correct.	
b. Develop auditory closure.	Present words, sound by sound, and have patient identify the word by either pointing to a picture of the word or saying the word. Increase gradually the length of the words and decrease the familiarity of the words.	Percent correct.	
	Present a part of the word and have the patient point to a picture of the word or complete the word. Increase gradually the length of the words and decrease the familiarity of the words.	Same as above.	
3. Improve visual perceptual skills.			
a. Develop visual	Present pairs of written words and have patient indicate whether the	Percent correct.	

Goal	Procedure	Measurement	Comments
discrimination.	words are the same or different. Increase gradually the similarity of the words, decrease the familiarity of the words, and increase length.		
b. Develop scanning and tracking skills.	Use scanning and tracking tasks (cancellation and trail-making activities) outlined under Attention: • Uses cues including red lines or tactile markers (velcro) at margins and/or ruler or index card under each line as necessary • Decrease cues gradually.	Percent correct, number and type of cues required, and/or time required to complete task.	
	Present functional materials (e.g., vending machine, phone book, dictionary) and have patient scan for specific information. Use above cues and decrease gradually.	Same as above.	
c. Develop visual closure skills.	Present partial pictures of objects and have patient match the partial picture to a complete one or name it.	Percent correct.	
	Present parts of letters or words and have patient match, read, or write the completed letter or word.	Same as above.	
d. Develop figure-ground discrimination skills.	Present letters, numbers, words, or pictured objects that are embedded within a visually distracting background and have patient identify the figure in the foreground.	Percent correct.	
e. Improve spatial relationship skills.	Present a series of shapes, letters, and numbers turned in different directions and have patient match the one that is similar to a target item. Increase gradually the number in the series and the degree of similarity between the target item and the foils.	Percent correct.	For some patients it is helpful to initially use cutout shapes, letters, and numbers that can be rotated so that the concept of spatial rotation is more concrete.

Goal	Procedure	Measurement	Comments
	Present a series of shapes, letters, and numbers, all of which are oriented in the same direction except for one, and have patient identify the one that is oriented differently. Increase gradually the number in the series and the degree of similarity between the target item and the foils.	Same as above.	
	Present a series of connecting lines oriented in different directions and overlaid on a grid of dots and have patient trace or copy (see Exhibit 5-10). Increase gradually the complexity of the design.	Percent/number of dots correctly connected and/or time taken to complete the task.	

Exhibit 5-10 Example of Visual-Spatial Relationship Exercise

Directions: Copy lines on each grid at left onto grid at right.

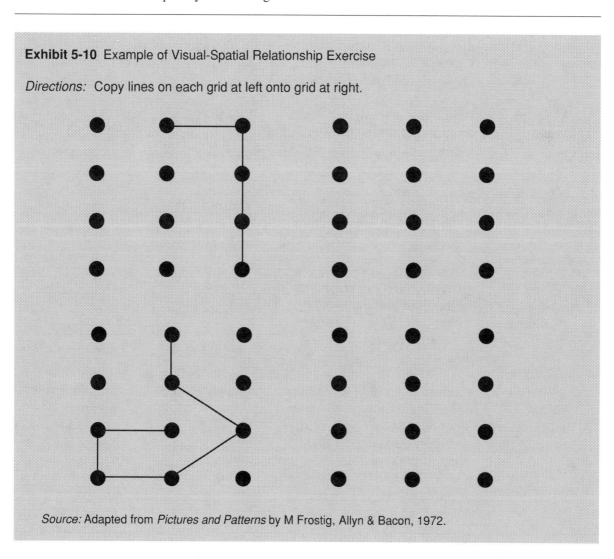

Source: Adapted from *Pictures and Patterns* by M Frostig, Allyn & Bacon, 1972.

PRAGMATICS/SEMANTICS

Impairment in the pragmatics of communication is a major problem in the traumatic brain injured patient and should be addressed throughout treatment. For example, while working on attentional activities such as attending to a speaker or shifting from one speaker to another, the speech-language pathologist is simultaneously working on improving eye contact. While facilitating orientation to person the clinician may also focus on developing awareness of specific idiosyncratic voice characteristics. While working on organization skills, the clinician can stress discourse organization and cohesion.

The treatment of pragmatic problems often can be conducted more effectively in a group setting, which permits more natural interactions. Videotapes are also a useful adjunct to treatment of pragmatics. For example, group interactions can be captured on videotape and replayed for the group members to analyze specific pragmatic behaviors. Videotaping can be incorporated into many of the activities described below.

Techniques typically used for dysarthria and voice problems, in addition to the procedures presented in this section may be applicable for the treatment of prosodic disturbances. Techniques for improving word retrieval deficits will not be addressed since they are available in the aphasia literature. Activities included in the section on the treatment of organization problems, particularly categorization, can facilitate improvement in semantic skills.

Goal	Procedure	Measurement	Comments
1. Improve comprehension and use of prosody.	Present a visual list of different communication intents (e.g., question, command, statement). Verbally present a sentence and have patient identify the intent (see Exhibit 5-11).	Percent correct.	
	Present a visual list of different emotions (e.g., anger, joy, surprise). Verbally present a sentence and have patient identify the intent of the sentence (see Exhibit 5-11).	Same as above.	
	Have patient repeat or spontaneously produce a sentence with specific communication intent or emotion.	Same as above.	
	Tape record the above and have patient identify whether the appropriate intent or emotion was conveyed.	Percent agreement between the patient and clinician.	
2. Improve comprehension and use of nonverbal			

Goal	Procedure	Measurement	Comments
communication behaviors.			
a. Eye contact.	Initiate a conversation with a second person in the treatment room (e.g., family member, another patient) and have patient shift eye contact to each new speaker: • Use exaggerated vocal inflection or gestures to help patient shift eye contact from speaker to speaker • Decrease gradually the use of the exaggerated cues as well as length of each speaker's turn.	Number of appropriate eye contact shifts per designated time period and/or type and number of cues required per shift.	See section on Attention.
	Use the above treatment procedure in group treatment with at least three patients. Increase gradually the number of patients in the group.	Same as above.	
b. Facial expression.	Present a photograph of (or clinician mimics) a facial expression. Have patient identify whether the facial expression in the photograph is positive or negative.	Percent correct.	
	Present a photograph of (or clinician mimics) a facial expression. Have patient match the expression to one of a list of situations (e.g., happy face to birthday party, contented face to having just finished a good meal).	Percent agreement between patient and clinician.	
	Present a given emotion or situation and have patient imitate or spontaneously produce the appropriate facial expression.	Same as above.	Body posture and gestures are used to augment interpretation and expression of emotions. However, for certain patients it may be necessary to focus on facial expressions first, and

Goal	*Procedure*	*Measurement*	*Comments*
			then add the other nonverbal behaviors. For other patients all these nonverbal behaviors should be used together to facilitate the interpretation and use of emotions.
c. Proxemics, body posture, gesture.	Assume a pose or present photographs that depict a designated attitude (e.g., anger, boredom, relaxation) and have patient identify it.	Percent correct.	
	Present a given attitude and have patient imitate or spontaneously assume the appropriate pose.	Same as above.	
d. All the above nonverbal communication behaviors.	Present in a group situation a specific emotion and have one patient provide the appropriate facial expression and pose. Ask the other patients to evaluate whether it is correct or incorrect.	Percent correct for patient performing the emotion and/or agreement between clinician and patients' evaluation of the pose.	
	Have patients identify the specific emotion presented by the clinician or another patient.	Percent agreement between clinician's and patients' evaluation of the emotion and/or percent agreement between designated emotion and performance by the patient.	
3. Improve conversational skills.			
a. Initiation of a conversation and topic selection.	Present patient with a topic and two statements. Have patient identify which one is the more appropriate introductory statement (see Exhibit 5-12).	Percent correct.	

Goal	Procedure	Measurement	Comments
	Present the patient with a topic and have patient give an appropriate introductory statement. Cue by providing an introductory statement for the patient to model.	Same as above.	
	Present a choice of topics and have patient select one and then provide an introductory statement for it.	Same as above.	
	Have patient initiate a topic and give an introductory statement. Cue with categories of topics as necessary.	Number of topics initiated, number of cues required, and/or percent of appropriate introductory statements.	
b. Topic maintenance.	Present a topic and an introductory statement and have patient maintain the topic for a designated period of time. Use verbal cues to redirect patient back to the topic.	Length of time patient maintains topic and number of cues.	
	Present a topic and have the patient introduce and maintain the topic for a designated period of time. Cue as above.	Same as above.	
c. Turn-taking.	Present a script of a conversation of two people and have patient identify whether or not the speakers took their turns appropriately (see Exhibit 5-13). • Cue with elaboration of meaning of the content and the sequencing of ideas by the speakers • Increase gradually the number of speakers in the script.	Percent correct and type and number of cues required.	For some patients who have difficulty interpreting nonverbal communication behaviors, this approach that focuses on content is useful.
	Present a videotape of a conversation of two people and have patient identify whether or not the speakers took their turns appropriately: • Cue with elaboration of meaning of the content, interpretation of nonverbal communication	Same as above.	

Goal	*Procedure*	*Measurement*	*Comments*
	behaviors and sequencing of ideas • Increase gradually the number of speakers.		
	Videotape a conversation between the patient and clinician and have patient identify whether or not the speakers took their turns appropriately. Cue as above as necessary.	Same as above.	
4. Improve the organization and completeness of discourse.			
a. Narrative discourse.	Present three pictures depicting a story and have patient sequence them in the correct order and then tell the story. Increase gradually the number of pictures.	Percent of pictures and utterances correctly ordered.	This activity is also appropriate for improving organizational skills.
	Present a short story auditorily or visually and have patient retell the story: • Cue with key words written sequentially and decrease as appropriate • Increase gradually the length of the story.	Percent of pertinent facts included, percent correctly ordered and number of cues.	This activity is also appropriate for improving memory.
	Have patient tell a story about a personal event.	Percent of relevant facts included and correctly ordered.	
	Audiotape or videotape or write down the patient's responses for any of the above narrative tasks. Have patient identify any incorrectly sequenced responses and then correct the sequence.	Percent of errors correctly identified and percent correctly resequenced.	
b. Procedural discourse.	Present out of sequence the written steps involved in performing a familiar task (e.g., getting dressed, making coffee, mailing a letter)	Percent correctly ordered.	

Goal	Procedure	Measurement	Comments
	and have patient sequence the steps in the correct order. Increase gradually the number of steps involved and the unfamiliarity of the task.		
	Present a familiar task and have patient explain the steps involved in performing the activity. Increase the complexity and unfamiliarity of the task.	Percent of pertinent facts included and correctly ordered.	These tasks can be used also for improving organizational skills.
c. Improve use of cohesive ties.	Present a short written narrative in which all pronouns and deictic terms are underlined and have patient identify the referent of each pronoun/deictic term (see Exhibit 5-14). Increase gradually the distance between the pronoun/ deictic term and its referent.	Percent correct.	
	Present a short written narrative and have patient delete information that is understood from the context (see Exhibit 5-15). Increase gradually the distance between the pairs of related ideas.	Same as above.	
	Present a narrative of short sentences and have patient select from a list the appropriate conjunctions to insert between related sentences (see Exhibit 5-16).	Same as above.	
	Audiotape, videotape or write down the patient's telling or retelling of a story and then have patient identify correct and incorrect use or absence of reference, ellipsis, and/or conjunctions.	Same as above.	

Exhibit 5-11 Types of Communication Intents and Emotions

COMMUNICATION INTENTS

Types of Intents:

Q = Question
C = Command
S = Statement

Sample Sentences with Multiple Meaning Dependent on Prosodic Variations:

1. You are going to the movie. (Q, C, S)
2. Sit down. (Q, C, S)
3. I am lost. (Q, S)
4. It's bedtime. (Q, C, S)
5. You have been invited to the party. (Q, S)
6. It is time to do homework. (Q, C, S)
7. He made you a job offer. (Q, S)
8. The towels are in the dryer. (Q, S)
9. Turn the television on to Channel 2. (Q, C)
10. You wash your hands before dinner. (C, S)

EMOTIONS

Types of Emotions:

A = Anger
D = Disgust
E = Excitement
H = Happiness/Joy
Sa = Sadness
Su = Surprise

Sample Sentences with Multiple Emotional Intents Dependent on Prosodic Variations:

1. I won a million dollars in the state lottery. (E, H, Su)
2. My best friend moved to New York. (A, D, E, H, Sa, Su)
3. He has a huge German Shepherd for a pet. (D, E, H, Su)
4. I really dislike it when you make a mess in the house. (A, D, Sa)
5. I have the flu for the third time this winter. (A, D, Sa, Su)
6. The repairs on the car cost 300 dollars. (A, D, H, Sa, Su)
7. She received a new television set for her birthday. (E, H, Su)
8. I've tried to reach her three times but there has been no answer. (A, D, Sa, Su)
9. We went to a Mexican restaurant for dinner on Saturday night. (A, D, E, H, Sa, Su)
10. You slipped on the ice again. (A, D, Sa, Su)

Exhibit 5-12 Selecting Appropriate Introductory Statements

Directions: From each pair of sentences, select the best statement to introduce the topic.

TOPIC: SPORTS

1. Did you watch the game last night?
2. The pitcher struck out in the third inning.

1. He hit the best lob I saw all night.
2. I enjoy playing tennis at least once a week.

TOPIC: RESTAURANTS

1. I went to a great new Chinese restaurant last night.
2. The chicken chow mein was too salty.

1. The french fries were so greasy.
2. I couldn't resist stopping at McDonald's on the way home.

TOPIC: WORK

1. I went for a job interview yesterday.
2. They did not offer me enough money for the position.

1. Finally I decided to go into computers.
2. What line of work are you in?

TOPIC: MOVIES

1. Then the scene switched back to the prison.
2. Did you see the new movie at the Main Street Theater?

1. I heard you saw a wonderful movie over the weekend.
2. I disagreed with what the critics said about it.

Exhibit 5-13 Identifying Appropriate Turn-Taking from a Script

Directions: Tell me whether each speaker has taken a turn at the right time.

SCRIPT 1

MARY: John, I'd like you to meet Ann Smith. Ann, this is my friend John Jones.
ANN: Hello, John.
JOHN: Hello, Ann. I have a sister named Ann. Do you spell your name A-n-n or A-n-n-e?
MARY: Where does your sister live?

SCRIPT 2

JOAN: I heard you went to a great sale yesterday.
LINDA: Yes, I did. It was at the new shopping mall.
JOAN: What did you buy?
LINDA: I bought four blouses, two skirts and . . .
JOAN: Did you go to the shoe store, too?
LINDA: And a nightgown with a matching robe. What else did you ask?

Exhibit 5-14 Identifying the Referents

Directions: Identify the noun that goes with each italicized word.

PARAGRAPH 1

Mrs. Brown gave her husband a shopping list. *He* went to the supermarket and spent 100 dollars *there*. *They* were very surprised at the cost.

PARAGRAPH 2

The president addressed the nation last night. *He* told *us* the economy has been steadily improving since the first of the year. *It* has risen over 10%. *We* were all surprised by *this*.

PARAGRAPH 3

Sharon and Bob went to a brand new restaurant. *It* had wonderful Italian food. *They* had minestrone soup, pasta, and garlic bread. The soup, pasta, and bread were tasty. *They* are going back *there* tomorrow.

Exhibit 5-15 Identifying Information that Can Be Deleted

Directions: Identify the words that can be deleted without changing the meaning of the paragraph.

PARAGRAPH 1

Mr. and Mrs. James are going to Washington, D.C. They are staying in Washington, D.C. for two weeks. The James are planning to see all the sights of Washington, D.C. The James' children will join them in Washington, D.C. after one week.

PARAGRAPH 2

Mrs. Jackson went to the pet store last weekend. She wanted to buy a puppy at the pet store. She ended up buying a black Cocker Spaniel at the pet store. She paid $40 for the puppy. She plans to surprise her son with the puppy.

Exhibit 5-16 Using Conjunctions to Connect Sentences

Directions: Select from the list the appropriate conjunctions to insert in the space between related sentences.

PARAGRAPH 1

Mr. and Mrs. James are going to Washington, D.C. _____ they are staying for two weeks. Their children are coming _____ they are staying for only one week.

and   because   but   so

PARAGRAPH 2

Mary takes piano lessons three times a week _____ she would prefer to take lessons every day. She hopes to be a concert pianist _____ travel all around the world performing. The teacher thinks she will succeed _____ she practices at least an hour each day.

and   because   but   so

MEMORY

There have been two basic approaches to the treatment of memory disorders.[1] The first is restoration which focuses on improving memory through the use of exercises and drills. However, only minimal improvement in functional memory has been demonstrated in traumatic brain injured patients utilizing this approach.[1] The second approach used in retraining memory is teaching the use of strategies to compensate for the memory loss.

There are primarily two types of compensatory strategies: external compensatory (e.g., calendar, clock, memory book); and internal facility (e.g., mnemonics, chunking, visual imagery). Treatment should stress the use of external compensatory strategies and the generalization of their use to the natural environment. In addition, internal facilitory strategies can be used for facilitating the retention of small amounts of specific information that is important to the patient.[1] The clinician should not expect the patient to spontaneously use the internal strategies functionally to recall large amounts of general information in the environment.

Our goals and procedures will primarily focus on developing the patient's awareness of the need to use compensatory strategies, identifying those specific strategies that will be useful to the patient, and facilitating the use of these strategies. A vital component of memory rehabilitation is the counseling of family members and other caregivers on how best to use these techniques with the patient. Further, the clinician should instruct the family on how to organize the patient's environment to maximize memory capabilities.

Goal	Procedure	Measurement	Comments
1. Develop awareness of the need to use compensatory strategies.	Provide a simple piece of information (e.g., where to go when treatment is completed or clinician's name) and instruct patient to remember the information: • Have patient recall the information after an interval of time that you know he/she would have forgotten it • Stress the idea that the patient forgot the information and point out that there are ways to assist in remembering.	Ratio of the number of times patient was aware information had not been remembered correctly to the number of times the information was actually forgotten.	This procedure is appropriate only for those patients who are unaware or deny that they have a memory problem. This activity will need to be repeated several times during the session and over a period of time.
2. Develop use of external compensatory strategies.	Present a memory book with the selected categories that are relevant to the patient's needs and level of functioning (see Exhibit 5-17). Cue with names of the categories. Have the patient: • Locate each of the named categories • Locate in which category specific information belongs • Retrieve specific information from the memory book.	Percent correct. Same as above. Percent of times patient referred to	

Goal	Procedure	Measurement	Comments
		memory book, accuracy of information retrieved, and number of cues required.	
	Present a list of weekly activities and have the patient write appointments in the appropriate section of a memory book, appointment book, or on a calendar.	Percent of information written in the correct section.	
	Present a situation (e.g., going shopping, planning a party, running errands) and have patient make a list of the pertinent items that will assist in completing the task.	Percent of correct information included on the list.	
	Present a task and the list of steps or items required to complete that task (e.g., making an appointment on the telephone, replying to an invitation): • Have patient complete the task while referring to the list • Cue patient to refer to the list as necessary.	Percent of steps correctly followed, number of times patient spontaneously referred back to the list and number of cues.	
	Present a task in writing and the time for initiating the task (e.g., open the door at 3:00 P.M.): • Have patient perform the task at the designated time • Cue patient to refer to a clock or watch • Increase gradually the time between presentation of the information and the initiation of the task, and the number and complexity of the intervening tasks.	Number of times task is performed at the designated time, number of intervening tasks, length of intervening period, and/or number of cues required.	
3. Develop internal, facilitatory strategies.	Identify specific information that is important for the patient to remember (e.g., names of siblings) and the appropriate strategy to facili-	Accuracy of recall of information, type and number of cues required, and length	

Goal	Procedure	Measurement	Comments
	tate the learning of this information (see Exhibit 5-18). <ul><li>Have patient learn the strategy and recall the specified information immediately, and after a specified interval of time</li><li>Cue by demonstration, use of drawing, and repetition.</li></ul>	of time information is retained.	
4. Develop use of directed listening or reading strategies to improve retention of auditory or visually presented information.	Present a visual or auditory message (e.g., phone message, instruction from the doctor) and have patient recall the information: <ul><li>Cue by directing the patient to listen or look for specific information</li><li>Increase gradually the length of the message and the number of salient points</li><li>Decrease gradually the amount of directed listening or reading cues.</li></ul>	Percent correct of key information retained and number of cues required.	
5. Use external compensatory and internal facilitatory strategies in a functional environment.	Have the patient apply any of the above compensatory strategies in a less structured situation such as group treatment, role playing a situation, or a supervised out-trip (e.g., grocery store, bank, post-office).	Number of times patient self-initiated an appropriate compensatory strategy or type and number of cues required to facilitate use of the strategy.	It is important to allow family members/ caregivers to observe and participate in these activities as an initial step to counseling and training.
	Counsel family members/ caregivers and staff to encourage the patient to use compensatory and facilitory strategies. Train them in the use of appropriate cuing techniques.	Family/caregiver and/or staff feedback.	
	Counsel family members/ caregivers, patient, and staff on ways to organize the environment to facilitate memory (e.g., a designated place for routinely used items, labels on drawers and cabinets).	Same as above.	

Exhibit 5-17 Suggested Categories for Memory Book

1. Demographic/biographical information
2. Calendar
3. Daily schedule
4. Significant people
5. Personal events/experiences
6. Treatment log
7. List of things to do
8. Current events
9. Work information

Exhibit 5-18 Internal Facilitory Strategies

REHEARSAL

Repetitive practice

- When first introduced to a new person, ask the person to spell or pronounce his name clearly and distinctly; repeat this several times during your initial conversation.

  Mary: "Hi! My name is Mary Peters."
  Patient: "Hi, Mary. My name is John. Mary, how do you spell Peters?

SALIENCY

Focus on the most important information within a message first and then the less meaningful information.

- When taking a telephone message, note the name and telephone number first; then complete the contextual information.
- When taking notes in a class, write dates and names before writing other contextual information.

CHUNKING

Create meaningful groups to enable more information to be retained at a given time.

- Phone number 864-3642 recalled as eight hundred sixty-four, thirty-six, forty-two.
- Six grocery items may be remembered better by chunking them into dairy products, meat, and vegetables.

MNEMONICS

Acronyms

Formulate a word from the first letter of items.

- Susan the speech-language pathologist = SOS = Susan of Speech.

Rhyme and Melody

Formulate a rhyme to link words.

- Ambulation = a heel and a toe and away we go.

IMAGERY

(Patients may vary in their ability to benefit from static versus action images.)

Retracing Events

Assist in the recall of previous occurrences.

- Look for lost keys by visualizing when you had them last and the activities following.
- Remember what was eaten for breakfast by visualizing the breakfast tray.

Conventional Images

Associate and relate interacting pairs of items.

- Mary Brown is married and has brown hair.
- Remembering the supermarket "Jewel" by visualizing a gemstone.

Absurd Images

Make a novel or ridiculous connection with an item.

- Mary Burns with her hair on fire.
- Mr. Lee with a Sara Lee pie on his face.

Out-of-Proportion Images

Visualize an aspect of an item as larger or smaller.

- The physical therapist associated with a large cane.
- The audiologist with huge ears.
- The doctor with six stethoscopes.

Out-of-Place Images

Associate an item in an unexpected place.

- To remember keys, visualize them next to the coffee pot.
- To remember to complete homework, visualize it taped over the television set.
- To remember to practice range of motion exercises, visualize the sling on top of the television set.

Source: Adapted from *Clinical Management of Right Hemisphere Dysfunction* (p 85) by MS Burns, AS Halper and SI Mogil (Eds), Aspen Publishers Inc, © 1985.

HIGHER LEVEL COGNITIVE PROCESSES: ORGANIZATION, REASONING, AND PROBLEM SOLVING/JUDGMENT

Although organization, reasoning, and problem solving/judgment are closely interrelated, the following procedures delineate treatment activities that target primarily one process at a time. However, real-life situations often require the integration of these three processes. Many of these procedures may be appropriate only for the more mildly involved patient. Furthermore, the patient's educational and vocational level and premorbid interests and cognitive abilities must be taken into consideration in the selection of any of these treatment activities.

Goal	Procedure	Measurement	Comments
1. Improve organization skills			
a. Categorization.	Present a series of geometric shapes using blocks and/or picture cards and have patient sort them by shape, color or size: • Start sorting by one feature (e.g., color only) and gradually increase the number of features (e.g., color and shape) • Cue by questioning the rationale for sorting the geometric shapes into a specific category.	Percent correct and/ or accuracy of rationale for sorting.	Although this task stresses sorting by perceptual features, it is useful for teaching the concept of categorization.
	Present a series of objects, picture cards or words and have patient sort them by semantic category (e.g., transportation versus animals): • Cue by questioning the rationale for sorting the items into a specific semantic category • Increase gradually the number of categories by which the item should be sorted as well as the similarity between the categories (land versus water vehicles).	Same as above.	
	Present a target word or picture and three other items, one of which is associated with the target. Have the patient match the latter item with the target (see Exhibit 5-19). • Cue by questioning the rationale	Percent correct and/ or accuracy of rationale for selection of associated items.	

Goal	Procedure	Measurement	Comments
	for the selection of the associated item • Increase gradually the number of foils and the similarity between the foils and the target (see Exhibit 5-19).		
	Present a list auditorily or visually of three items and have patient select the one that does not belong: • Cue by questioning the rationale for the selection of the target item • Increase gradually the number of items and the similarity between the target and foils.	Percent correct and/or accuracy of rationale for selection of target items.	
	Present functional topics and have patient sort items into the appropriate categories (see Exhibit 5-20). Cue by questioning the rationale for sorting the item into a specific category.	Percent correct and/or accuracy of rationale for sorting.	
	Present pairs of words auditorily or visually and have patient explain how the items are alike and different (e.g., car/airplane): • Increase gradually the similarity of the items (e.g., car/bus) • Increase gradually the number of similarities and differences the patient is required to give.	Percent correct.	
	Present an analogy task visually or auditorily and have patient provide the target response (e.g., apple is to fruit as lettuce is to ____): • Use a variety of relationships such as opposites, synonyms, part-whole relationships, and function • Cue by questioning the relationship between the analogous pair of words.	Percent correct and/or accuracy of rationale given.	This task requires the ability to reason inductively.
b. Sequencing.	Present the following and have patient sequence:	Percent correct.	

Goal	Procedure	Measurement	Comments
	• Letters of the alphabet • Letters into words • Words alphabetically • Words into sentences • Sentences into paragraphs • Pictures into activities • Paragraphs into stories • Steps for daily or familiar activities • Steps for less familiar activities (e.g., moving, taking a trip).		
	Present a sequence of words and have patient arrange the words in the correct order (e.g., foot, inch, yard). Cue by questioning the rationale for sequencing the items.	Percent correct, number of cues and/ or accuracy of rationale for sequencing.	
	Present a sequence of words and have patient complete the sequence (e.g., inch, foot, _____). Cue by providing several words for the patient to choose from (yard, pound, leg) or by providing the rationale for sequencing the item.	Percent correct and/ or type and number of cues.	
c. Prioritizing.	Present a situation (e.g., running errands, going shopping, preparing a household budget, planning a picnic), provide details or have patient itemize details. Have patient prioritize in order of importance or other salient features (e.g., time constraints, geographic location).	Number of details included and/or percent of agreement between the patient and the clinician.	The clinician can change the criteria for prioritizing the details and/or increase the number of criteria by which the patient reorders (see Exhibit 5-21).
d. Outlining.	Present two topics and a number of points related to each topic and have patient assign each point to the appropriate topic. Increase gradually the number of topics and/or points presented and the degree of similarity between the topics.	Percent correct.	
	Present a list of words or ideas and have patient organize into an	Percent correctly ordered and number	

Goal	Procedure	Measurement	Comments
	outline form with main topics and subtopics.	of cues required.	
	Present a paragraph visually and have patient identify: • the main idea • subtopics • details. Cue with questions and/or provide a partially completed or blank outline for the specific information given (see Exhibit 5-22). Increase gradually the number of paragraphs and the number of subtopics and details included.	Percent correct and number and type of cues required.	
	Present information auditorily or visually and have patient take notes enumerating the salient points.	Percent of salient facts included and/or percent correctly ordered.	
	Present a topic or situation or have patient initiate one. Have patient prepare an outline for a speech, letter, or memo.	Percent of pertinent facts included and/or percent correctly ordered.	
2. Improve reasoning skills. a. Inductive reasoning.	Present the following inductive reasoning tasks and have patient complete: • Inferences • Analogies • Cause and effect relationships • Identification of relevant information • Story completion. Cue with appropriate strategies for task completion and gradually decrease.	Percent correct, number of cues provided by the clinician, and/or number of self-initiated strategies generated.	
b. Deductive reasoning.	Present the following deductive reasoning tasks and have patient complete: • Determination of valid conclusions	Percent correct, number of cues provided by the clinician, and/or number of self-	

Goal	Procedure	Measurement	Comments
	• Identification of missing premises • Identification of a situation from detailed information • Mindbenders • Syllogisms. Cue with appropriate strategies and gradually decrease.	initiated strategies generated.	
c. Interpretation and appreciation of humor.	Present the following materials and have patient explain the humor: • Jokes • Amusing anecdotes • Puns • Cartoons and political satire.	Accuracy of rationale for humor.	
3. Improve problem solving and judgment skills.	Present a problem situation (e.g., fire, personal hazard) and have patient explain a possible response to the situation: • Encourage the patient to give more than one response to the situation • Cue with "wh" questions.	Percent of agreement between the clinician and the patient.	
	Present a problem situation with several alternative solutions and have patient: • Predict the consequences of each solution • Evaluate which solution is best and why.	Number of times patient is able to support his responses.	
	Present a situation involving two people (e.g., Mary goes to a party and finds that the hostess is wearing the same dress) and have patient explain how each person feels and why.	Number of times patient is able to support responses.	
	Present a situation or issue (e.g., the merits of a political candidate, lovelorn columns and editorials) and have patient delineate the advantages and disadvantages of each side.	Percent of agreement between the clinician and patient.	

Exhibit 5-19 Associations

Directions: Select the word (picture) that is best associated with the given word (picture).

FOOT	car	dog	leg
LION	apple	tiger	chair

INCREASING SIMILARITY OF FOILS

FOOT	wrist	eye	leg
LION	dog	canary	tiger

INCREASING SIMILARITY AND NUMBER OF FOILS

FOOT	knee	calf	heel	thigh
LION	elephant	gorilla	leopard	zebra

Exhibit 5-20 Suggested Functional Topics for Organization Activities

Book Titles (e.g., cookbooks, fiction, travel)

Grocery Items or Coupons (e.g., dairy products, canned goods, paper goods)

Records (e.g., jazz, classical, rock)

Magazines (e.g., fashion, home, news)

Movies (e.g., musicals, comedy, science fiction)

Newspaper Headlines, Captions, Pictures (e.g., sports, business, editorials)

Recipes (e.g., appetizers, soups, desserts)

Restaurants (e.g., Mexican, Italian, American)

Stores (e.g., shoes, toys, jewelry)

Television Programs (e.g., comedy, detective stories, news)

Exhibit 5-21 Change in Criteria for Prioritizing Information

EXAMPLE 1: Running Errands—Prioritize by geographic location.
Hardware store on 600 North Clark Street
Grocery store on 200 North State Street
Bakery on 780 North Clark Street
Dry cleaners at 430 North Clark Street
Drugstore on 333 North State Street

EXAMPLE 2: Running Errands—Prioritize by order of importance to prepare a dinner party.
Hardware store to pick up a hammer
Grocery store to buy meat, vegetables, and fruit
Bakery to buy dessert
Dry cleaners to pick up table cloth and napkins
Drugstore to buy a new toothbrush

EXAMPLE 3: Running Errands—Prioritize by budgetary constraints of $50 and run as many errands as possible.
Hardware store—$7.50
Grocery store—$45.00
Bakery—$20.00
Dry cleaners—$10.00
Drugstore—$12.00

Exhibit 5-22 Outlining

Directions: Read the following paragraphs and identify the main ideas, subtopics, and details. Fill in the appropriate spaces on the outline below.

Last month, 20,000 people participated in the Third Annual Chicago Marathon. The men's division was won by Ronald Carter, 22 years of age, from Moline, Illinois. He finished in two hours, eight minutes, and three seconds. This broke the Chicago Marathon record set last year by Robert Sells, but fell short of the world record.

Terry Turner, age 27, from Toronto, Canada won the women's division. She finished in two hours, 24 minutes, and 54 seconds. This was Ms. Turner's second victory this year.

This month an anticipated 25,000 will run in the 25th Annual New York Marathon. Both Ms. Turner and Mr. Carter will compete in this race. However, the favorites for the men's division are Carl Good and Jim Jones, both from Australia. The favorites for the women's division are two Americans, Gail Cooke and Jill Thomas.

TITLE: MARATHON RUNNING

I. _____ (Name of Marathon)

   A. Introduction

      1. _____ (When it Occurred)

      2. _____ (Number of Participants)

   B. Men's Division Winner

      1. _____ (Name)

      2. _____ (Where From)

      3. _____ (Age)

      4. _____ (Finishing Time)

   C. Women's Division Winner

      1. _____ (Name)

      2. _____ (Where From)

      3. _____ (Age)

      4. _____ (Finishing Time)

II. _____ (Name of Marathon)

   A. Introduction

      1. _____ (When it Occurred)

      2. _____ (Number of Participants)

   B. Men's Favorites

      1. _____ (Name and Where From)

      2. _____ (Name and Where From)

   C. Women's Favorites

      1. _____ (Name and Where From)

      2. _____ (Name and Where From)

CONCLUSION

In summary, we have presented goals, procedures, and measures for the treatment of cognitive-linguistic problems in the traumatic brain injured adult. We have discussed sensory stimulation techniques as well as treatment for each of the processes of attention, perception, orientation, semantics/pragmatics, memory, organization, reasoning, and problem solving/judgment. It is essential that the speech-language pathologist understand the underlying processes that are impacting on effective communication and executive functioning. The suggestions given are intended as a treatment guide to aid the clinician in choosing appropriate goals, carrying out a treatment program, and measuring and documenting progress. They must be carefully adapted and applied to the individual patient.

REFERENCES

1. Sohlberg MM, Mateer C. *Introduction to Cognitive Rehabilitation.* New York, NY: Guilford Press; 1989.
2. Ylvisaker M, Szekeres SF, Henry K, Sullivan DM, Wheeler P. Topics in cognitive rehabilitation therapy. In: Ylvisaker M, Gobble EMRF, eds. *Community Re-entry for Head Injured Adults.* Boston, Mass: College-Hill Press; 1987:137–220.
3. Smith GJ, Ylvisaker M. Cognitive rehabilitation therapy: early stages of recovery. In: Ylvisaker M, ed. *Head Injury: Children and Adolescents.* Boston, Mass: College-Hill Press; 1985:275–286.
4. Moore JC. Neuroanatomic considerations relating to recovery of function following brain lesions. In: Bach-y-Rita, P, ed. *Recovery of Function: Theoretical Considerations for Brain Injury.* Gaithersburg, Md: Aspen Publishers Inc; 1980:9–90.
5. Farber SD. *Neurorehabilitation: A Multisensory Approach.* Philadelphia, Pa: WB Saunders Co; 1982.
6. Burns MS, Halper AS, Mogil SI. Diagnosis of communication problems in right hemisphere damage. In: Burns MS, Halper AS, Mogil SI, eds. *Clinical Management of Right Hemisphere Damage.* Gaithersburg, Md: Aspen Publishers Inc; 1985:29–56.
7. Szekeres SF, Ylvisaker M, Cohen SB. A framework for cognitive rehabilitation therapy. In: Ylvisaker M, Gobble EMRF, eds. *Community Re-entry for Head Injured Adults.* Boston, Mass: College-Hill Press; 1987: 87–136.

Commercially Available Treatment Materials

KEY

Process

A   = Attention
M   = Memory
ORG = Organization
O   = Orientation
P   = Perception
PR = Pragmatics
PJ = Problem Solving/Judgment
R   = Reasoning
S   = Semantics
*   = Adaptable for use within designated area

	A	M	ORG	O	P	PR	PJ	R	S
						Process			

Alemany Press
2501 Industrial Parkway West
Hayward CA 94545

The Action Reporter by Armando Riverol.
  Consists of exercises using formats newspaper reporters routinely use in interviewing and reporting. — PR ✔, PJ *

All Sides of the Issue: Activities for Cooperative Jigsaw Groups by Elizabeth Coelho, Lisa Winer, and Judy Winn-Bell Olsen.
  Contains readings presenting socially important issues such as the law, immigration, and environmental pollution from four distinctive points of view. — PR ✔, PJ ✔, R ✔

Business Telephone Skills by Carolyn Feuille-Le Chevallier.
  Consists of exercises and activities to develop effective business telephone skills. — PR ✔

| | | | | Process | | | | |
A	M	ORG	O	P	PR	PJ	R	S

Decisions by Barbara Bowers and John Godfrey.

Consists of open-ended problems presented in anecdotal form with possible solutions focusing on such issues as local agencies offering legal advice and organizations dealing with consumer complaints.

Decisions, Decisions by Barbara Bowers and John Godfrey.

Consists of open-ended problems presented in anecdotal form with possible solutions focusing on such issues as the difference between a line of credit, a personal loan, a mortgage, and the legal requirements for a day care center.

Functioning in English by David Mendelsohn, Rose Laufer, and Jura Seskus.

Consists of activities that provide practice and discussion for such communicative interactions as expressing likes and dislikes, persuading, and requesting and giving information and directions.

Partners 1, 2, 3 by Michael Lewis.

Contains information-gap problem situations to be resolved through communicating with a partner.

What's So Funny by Elizabeth Claire.

Consists of activities focusing on understanding humor and telling jokes.

Allied Educational Press
P.O. Box 337
Niles, MI 49120

The Fitzhugh Plus Program by Kathleen Fitzhugh and Loren Fitzhugh.

"Book 101: Shape Matching"
Contains exercises for figure rotation, size variations, and matching similar and exact shapes.

"Book 102: Shape Completion"
Contains exercises that focus on such areas as visual motor-memory and completion of shapes.

"Book 104: Shape Analysis and Sequencing"
Contains exercises that focus on such areas as fig-

Entry	A	M	ORG	O	P	PR	PJ	R	S
Decisions						✔	✔	✔	
Decisions, Decisions							✔	✔	
Functioning in English						✔	✔	✔	
Partners 1, 2, 3						✔	✔		
What's So Funny						✔		✔	
Book 101: Shape Matching					✔				
Book 102: Shape Completion					✔				
Book 104: Shape Analysis and Sequencing					✔			✔	

	A	M	ORG	O	P	PR	PJ	R	S
Process									

ure analysis, figure-ground differentiation, and figure interpretation and memory.

Barnell Loft Ltd.
958 Church Street
Baldwin, NY 11510

Developing Key Concepts in Comprehension: Books E-H, Advanced 1 by Richard Boning.
   Contains exercises targeting narration, cause and effect, definition, description, problem-solution, and referencing.

	A	M	ORG	O	P	PR	PJ	R	S
Developing Key Concepts		*				✔	✔	✔	✔

Multiple Skills Series: Books E-I by Richard Boning.
   Contains written paragraphs followed by questions addressing the main idea, details, inferences, and vocabulary (Spanish Edition available).

	A	M	ORG	O	P	PR	PJ	R	S
Multiple Skills		*						✔	✔

Specific Skill Series: Books G-L
   Contains exercises focusing on getting the main idea, drawing conclusions, using the context, following directions, detecting the sequence, and identifying inferences.
   "Detecting the Sequence" by Richard Boning.
   "Drawing Conclusions" by Richard Boning.
   "Following Directions" by Richard Boning.
   "Getting the Facts" by Richard Boning.
   "Getting the Main Idea" by Richard Boning.
   "Identifying Inferences" by William Wittenberg.
   "Locating the Answer" by Richard Boning.
   "Using the Context" by Richard Boning.

	A	M	ORG	O	P	PR	PJ	R	S
Specific Skill Series	✔	✔						✔	

Supportive Reading Skills: Sets E, F, Advanced by Richard Boning.
   Contains exercises that focus on such areas as comprehension, vocabulary, survival, and study skills.
   "Mastering Multiple Meanings"
   "Interpreting Idioms"
   "Reading Schedules"
   "Reading Ads"
   "Using a Table of Contents"
   "Using an Index"

	A	M	ORG	O	P	PR	PJ	R	S
Supportive Reading Skills		✔		✔				✔	✔

Charles C. Thomas Publishers
2600 South First Street
Springfield, IL 62794-9265

	Process							
A	M	ORG	O	P	PR	PJ	R	S

The Thinking Skills Workbook: A Cognitive Skills Remediation Manual for Adults, 2nd ed. by Lynn Tondat Carter, John L. Carsuso, and Mary A. Languirand.

Contains such exercises as visual scanning for letters and words, recalling pictures and numbers, matching geometric forms, reading maps, and categorizing words.

A	M	ORG	O	P	PR	PJ	R	S
✔	✔	✔	✔	✔			✔	

Communication Skill Builders
P.O. Box 42050
Tucson, AZ 85733

Activities and Ideas: Games for Adult and Adolescent Communication Groups by Janet D. Bisset and Mary Sue Fino.

Contains exercises such as providing synonyms, word associations, categorization, and sequencing tasks.

A	M	ORG	O	P	PR	PJ	R	S
		✔						✔

Cause and Effect Card Games: Social Judgment Skills for Head Injured Adolescents and Adults by Karen Bradley Richards and Maureen O'Brien Fallon.

Consists of games utilizing real life situations that cover such concerns as drinking, drugs, and hygiene.

A	M	ORG	O	P	PR	PJ	R	S
					✔	✔	✔	

Do You Remember When.

Contains five sets of photographs depicting people, activities, events, and other important features for each decade from the twenties through the sixties.

A	M	ORG	O	P	PR	PJ	R	S
	*				*	*		

Focus on Function: Retraining for the Communicatively Impaired Client by Shelly C. Hahn and Evelyn Klein.

Consists of a complete kit of evaluation forms, task cards, picture cards, and manipulatives stressing functional communication skills such as using the phone directory, making appointments, and using checks and money.

A	M	ORG	O	P	PR	PJ	R	S
	✔	✔	✔		*	✔		

Group Treatment for Head Injury: A Linguistic and Cognitive Approach by Marjorie Feinstein-Whittaker and Eileen O'Connell-Goodfellow.

Contains guidelines, exercises, and record keeping forms in the areas of augmentative communication,

A	M	ORG	O	P	PR	PJ	R	S
	✔	✔			✔	✔	✔	

	Process							
A	M	ORG	O	P	PR	PJ	R	S

verbal reasoning and problem solving, critical listening, and social discourse.

In Years Past
Contains nostalgic photographs of technology, transportation, events, famous people, fashion, and occupations.

A	M	ORG	O	P	PR	PJ	R	S
	*	*			*	*		

Pictures, Please! Adult Language Supplement by Marcia Stevenson Abbate and Elaine Fogel Schneider.
Consists of illustrations of persons, objects, or events for activities such as story telling and cause-effect.

A	M	ORG	O	P	PR	PJ	R	S
		✔			✔	✔	✔	

Problem Solving, Planning and Organizing Tasks: Strategies for Retraining by Vicki S. Parker and Nancy L. TenBroek.
Contains activities graded by complexity and organized into three areas: problem solving; planning and organization; and community-home assignments.

A	M	ORG	O	P	PR	PJ	R	S
		✔			✔	✔	✔	

The Question Collection: Teaching Questioning Strategies—A Pragmatic Approach by Ann Marquis and Elaine D. Trout.
Consists of a collection of card games including tasks such as formulating wh-questions, interpreting and making indirect requests, and role playing relevant life experiences.

A	M	ORG	O	P	PR	PJ	R	S
		✔			✔	✔	✔	

Questions for Thinking Skills: A Guided-Language Approach to Problem Solving by Monica Gustafson and Margaret Owen.
Consists of 50 photocards with guided questions to facilitate extracting information from pictures and manipulating it into new ideas.

A	M	ORG	O	P	PR	PJ	R	S
						✔	✔	

Reality Orientation: Principles and Practices by Lorna Rimmer.
Contains activities to help patients relearn basic facts about themselves and their environment.

A	M	ORG	O	P	PR	PJ	R	S
✔			✔					

Social Sequences
Contains six- to nine-card picture sequences of everyday activities such as making an omelet, going to the hairdresser, and taking a bath.

A	M	ORG	O	P	PR	PJ	R	S
			✔					

				Process					
	A	M	ORG	O	P	PR	PJ	R	S
Word Cues: Therapy for Retrieval by Jan Johnson.		✔							✔
Basic Life Skills by Jack Cassidy.	*	*						✔	
Connections: Working with Analogies: Levels C-F by Anthony Daniels.		✔						✔	✔
Reading for Comprehension: Junior High Edition by Thomas Gunning.	✔						✔	✔	
New Reading-Thinking Skills: Grades 3–6 by Ethel Maney and Anne Kroehler.		✔						✔	✔
Critical Steps To Effective Reading and Writing by Zenobia Verner and Bill Minturn.		✔					✔	✔	

Word Cues: Therapy for Retrieval by Jan Johnson.

Consists of a pocketbook that is carried by the patient and a clinician's manual with developmentally sequenced matching, sorting, and labeling activities.

The Continental Press, Inc.
520 East Bainbridge Street
Elizabeth, PA 17022

Basic Life Skills by Jack Cassidy.

Contains exercises that provide information on everyday activities such as job application and money-handling skills, followed by questions.

Connections: Working with Analogies: Levels C-F by Anthony Daniels.

Contains graduated tasks ranging from recognizing a given relationship to replicating it and then to generating original analogies of the same type.

Reading for Comprehension: Junior High Edition by Thomas Gunning.

Contains exercises for critical reading comprehension with questions that focus on assessing factual recall, determining meaning through context, completing analogies, making inferences, recognizing facts and opinions, and understanding multiple meanings.

New Reading-Thinking Skills: Grades 3–6 by Ethel Maney and Anne Kroehler.

Contains exercises focusing on such areas as inferences, organization of ideas, relationships, classifications, and meaning.

DLM
P.O. Box 4000
One DLM Park
Allen, TX 75002

Critical Steps To Effective Reading and Writing by Zenobia Verner and Bill Minturn.

Contains progressively structured reading exercises with questions that pertain to selecting the key idea, indicating the order of events, identifying cause and effect, distinguishing fact and opinion, and drawing conclusions.

	Process								
	A	M	ORG	O	P	PR	PJ	R	S
Independent-Living Sequential Cards. Consists of sequential picture cards depicting men and women doing household work such as the laundry, vacuuming, and dusting.			✔			✳			
Dormac, Inc. P.O. Box 270459 San Diego, CA 92128-0983									
Classics in Photostories by Lillian Butovsky and Cheryl Creatore. Consists of a three book series with audiocassettes dramatizing the photostory and discussion and listening activities.						✳			
Dormac Idiom Series by Myra Shulman Auslin. Consists of exercises covering: the definition of the idiom; application of the idiom to a given situation; vocabulary development; comprehension of the idiom; and the application of the idiom to personal experiences.							✔	✔	✔
In Other Words by Kathleen A. Santopietro. Consists of activities that require everyday problem solving on topics such as money and banking, transportation, and personal information.						✳	✔		
Many Meanings by Suzanne Dedrick and James Lattyak. Consists of three workbooks involving the understanding and correct usage of multiple meaning words.								✔	✔
Out of This World by Myra Shulman Auslin. Consists of exercises for idiom definitions, idiom comprehension, idiom application, and vocabulary development.								✔	✔
Simple English Classics adapted by Elizabeth V. DiSomma and Mary Louise McTiernan. Consists of works of classical fiction that have been written in simple English sentence structures with such exercises as sequencing, drawing conclusions, and answering various types of questions about the story.	✔	✔						✔	

				Process				
A	*M*	*ORG*	*O*	*P*	*PR*	*PJ*	*R*	*S*

Sticky Situations by Julia Jolly.

    Consists of realistic dilemmas encountered in school that require practical decision making. [PR ✶] [PJ ✔] [R ✔]

Time Concept Series by James Lattyak and Suzanne Dedrick.

    Consists of five workbooks presenting the concepts of day, week, month, season, and year through a variety of activities. [O ✔]

Vocabulary Building Exercises for the Young Adult by Dorothy McCarr.

    Consists of seven workbooks with activities such as unscrambling words and sentences, alphabetizing, and using the dictionary. [M ✔] [S ✔]

Educational Activities, Inc.
P.O. Box 392
Freeport, NY 11520

Developing Critical Thinking: Levels 3–6 by Eunice Insel and Ann Edson.

    Consists of problems which provide analytic reasoning practice in such situations as determining the proper sequence for doing research at the library and inferring logical answers from reading brief paragraphs. An audiocassette accompanies each book. [A ✶] [M ✔] [PJ ✔] [R ✔]

Listening and Notemaking Skills by Avis Agin and Johanna Prather.

    Consists of activity books and audiocassettes focusing on listening to a lecture, grasping the main and supporting ideas, and outlining. [A ✔] [M ✔]

Math for Everyday Living by Allen Schwartz and Anne R. Edson.

    Contains activities focusing on handling daily expenses, managing your money, and using math on the job. [O ✔] [PJ ✔]

EBSCO Curriculum Materials
Division of EBSCO Industries, Inc
P.O. Box 11521
Birmingham, AL 35201

					Process				
	A	M	ORG	O	P	PR	PJ	R	S
The Video Guide to Interviewing Series by Phil Mattox. Consists of three videos on the topics of preparing for an interview, handling difficult questions, and the four stages of interviewing.						*			
Educators Publishing Service, Inc. 75 Moulton Street Cambridge, MA 02138-1104									
Analogies 1, 2, 3 by Arthur Liebman. Contains activities for practicing analogy problems.								✔	✔
The Elements of Clear Thinking by William F. McCart.									
"Accurate Communication" Contains exercises for the use and misuse of language including positive and negative connotation, ambiguity, and triteness.					✔			✔	✔
"Critical Reasoning" Contains exercises focusing on such areas as outlining, paraphrasing, evaluating materials, and judging conclusions.			✔				✔	✔	
"Sound Reasoning" Contains instructions, examples and exercises on distinguishing between good and bad arguments of varying lengths and types.								✔	
Learning to Listen by William F. McCart. Contains exercises focusing on eight basic listening skills: following directions, following a sequence, using context clues, using different skills for different subject matter, finding topics and main ideas, listening for details, listening to make inferences, and taking notes while listening.	✔	✔						✔	
Reasoning and Reading: Levels 1, 2 by Joanne Carlisle. Contains activities focusing on part-whole relationships, finding categories, analogies, key words and generalizations, cause and effect, and syllogisms.			✔					✔	✔

	Process								
	A	M	ORG	O	P	PR	PJ	R	S
Reasoning and Reading by Joanne Carlisle.									
"Reasoning Skills 1, 2" Contains exercises for discriminating between fact and opinion, identifying relevant information, and drawing inferences.							✔	✔	
"Sentence Meaning 1, 2" Contains activities focusing on recognizing the main idea and the relationships between ideas.			✔					✔	✔
"Word Meaning 1, 2" Contains activities which focus on the relationships between words such as discriminating between good, vague, and imprecise definitions.								✔	✔
Wordly Wise: Books 7–9 by Kenneth Hodkinson and Joseph G. Ornato. Contains exercises dealing with analogies, connotations, and literal and metaphorical usage.								✔	✔
Fearon Education 500 Harbor Boulevard Belmont, CA 94002									
Budgeting by Charles Klasky. Contains activities focusing on short- and long-term budgeting and finances.			✔				*		
Buying with Sense by Carol L. King. Contains activities focusing on making consumer decisions, drawing up a budget, and finding a job.			✔				✔		
Checking Account by Daniel M. Finn. Contains step-by-step instructions about opening and maintaining a checking account and exercises such as filling out bank forms and check registers and writing checks.			✔						
Finding Your Way by Sally Grimes Pasley and Dee Koppel Williams. Contains exercises such as finding street addresses, recognizing landmarks, using taxicabs and subways, and interpreting maps and map symbols.				✔					

| | | | | *Process* | | | | |
A	M	ORG	O	P	PR	PJ	R	S

Forms by Nancy Anderton.
Contains 13 real job, bank and consumer forms.

| | ✔ | | | | | | | |

Give Me a Call by William Lefkowitz.
Contains activities that focus on taking down clear and legible messages, handling difficult incoming calls, determining the cost of a call, and using a map to determine the time zone of a particular state.

| | | ✔ | | ✔ | | ✔ | |

Lifetimes I, II by Tana Reiff.
Contains stories of real life experiences, such as dealing with alcoholism, choosing between family and career, and overusing a credit card, followed by questions.

| | ✱ | | | | ✔ | ✔ | ✔ | |

Mark Your Calendar by Sally Grimes Pasley and Dee Koppel Williams.
Contains activities focusing on basic calendar concepts and skills.

| | | | ✔ | | | | | |

Taking a Trip by Sally Grimes Pasley and Dee Koppel Williams.
Contains activities such as writing for travel information, deciding upon a destination, studying maps and schedules, and making reservations.

| | | | ✔ | | ✱ | ✱ | | |

Time and Telling Time by Bertha M. Wiley.
Contains exercises and activities focusing on clocks and telling time.

| | | | ✔ | | | | | |

Janus Books
2501 Industrial Parkway, West
Dept. K
Hayward, CA 94545

Action Sequence Stories: ACT II by Constance Olivia Williams.
Contains sequence cards centered around relevant situations. A resource book entitled "Interaction" supplements the cards and promotes discussion, role-playing, and imaginative thinking.

| | | ✔ | | | ✔ | | | |

Getting Around Cities and Towns by Winifred Ho Roderman.
Contains exercises such as how to get around one's own neighborhood, and reading building directories, street map, and bus routes.

| | | ✔ | ✔ | ✔ | | | | |

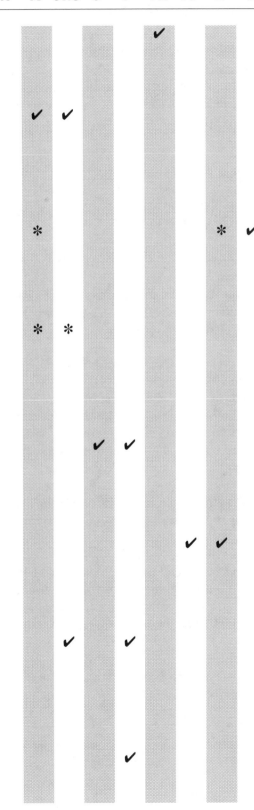

	Process								
	A	M	ORG	O	P	PR	PJ	R	S
Janus Job Interview Practice Pak by Wing Jew, Robert Tong and William Lefkowitz. Contains activities to simulate and role play job interviews.						✔			
Reading and Following Directions by Winifred Ho Roderman. Contains exercises that progress from simple, one-step directions to directions with two or more steps about such topics as using appliances, cooking, and assembling things.	✔	✔							
Our Government in Action by Richard Uhlich and William Lefkowitz. Contains short, focused units about such topics as the government, its history, and the U.S. Constitution, followed by comprehension and discussion questions.	✳							✳	✔
Reading a Newspaper by Phyllis Larned and Nicholas J. Randall. Contains activities for learning how to identify main news story ideas and supporting details, locating informative and entertaining features, and reading advertising.	✳	✳							
Reading Schedules by Winifred Ho Roderman. Contains activities for learning about different kinds of schedules and how to read them as well as how to understand abbreviations on calendars, bus schedules, class schedules, and movie/TV listings.				✔	✔				
Solving Word Problems by Susan D. Echaore and Winifred Ho Roderman. Consists of exercises such as analyzing word problems, extracting relevant facts, and estimating answers.							✔	✔	
Using the Phone Book by Patricia Gundlach and Keenan Kelsey. Contains activities for teaching applied alphabetical-order skills, clues to finding a phone number, how to use the yellow pages, and what is found in the index.				✔	✔				
Using the Want Ads by Wing Jew and Carol Tandy. Contains activities for learning to use the classified ad section.					✔				

				Process					
	A	*M*	*ORG*	*O*	*P*	*PR*	*PJ*	*R*	*S*

Understanding Word Problems by Mary Friedland and Winifred Ho Roderman.

Consists of activities for identifying basic parts of a word problem, using strategies to help solve problems, recognizing irrelevant information, and determining when two or more operations are needed.

		✔	✔			

LinguiSystems
3100 4th Avenue
P.O. Box 747
East Moline, IL 61244

ACE (Advanced Communication Exercises) by Kathryn J. Tomlin.

Contains such exercises as general information questions, question formulation, categorization, analogies, and stating opinions.

A ✔	*M* ✔					*PJ* ✔	*R* ✔	*S* ✔

Cognitive Connection by Maureen O'Connor and Pamela Vorce.

Consists of picture-stimuli illustrating problem situations and possible solutions with emphasis on predicting outcomes, explaining inferences, determining single and multiple causes and solutions, preventing and avoiding problems, and generalizing.

					PR ✳	*PJ* ✔	*R* ✔	

HELP (Handbook of Exercises for Language Processing) by Andrea M. Lazzari.

"HELP 1"
Contains exercises such as discriminating sounds and words, giving antonyms, determining likenesses and differences, and repeating numbers, words, and sentences.

A ✔	*M* ✔	*ORG* ✔		*P* ✔				*S* ✔

"HELP 2"
Contains exercises for categorization and answering wh-questions.

		ORG ✔					*R* ✔	*S* ✔

"HELP 3"
Contains exercises for identifying and describing relationships, paraphrasing sentences and paragraphs, solving problems, and developing pragmatic skills.

		ORG ✔			*PR* ✔	*PJ* ✔	*R* ✔	*S* ✔

	A	M	ORG	O	P	PR	PJ	R	S
				Process					
"HELP 4" Contains such exercises as identifying humor, explaining idioms, giving similarities and differences, and sorting items by attributes.		✔						✔	✔
HELP 1 & 2 Language Game by Andrea M. Lazzari and Patricia M. Peters. Consists of a board and dice game for one to four players. Question cards cover the same areas as in *HELP 1 & 2* handbooks with the addition of turn taking skills.	✔	✔	✔		✔	✔		✔	✔
HELP 3 & 4 Language Game by Andrea M. Lazzari and Patricia M. Peters. Consists of a Jeopardy-like game with questions that cover the same areas as in HELP 3 & 4.			✔			✔	✔	✔	✔
Just for Adults: An Adult Handbook for Language Rehabilitation by Andrea M. Lazzari. Consists of exercises such as evaluating information, explaining and correcting verbal absurdities, and identifying desirable characteristics of a person or object.		✔					✔	✔	
MEER and MEER Images by Linda Zachman, Rosemary Huisingh, Mark Barrett, Mary Kay Snedden, and Carol Jorgensen. Contains exercises such as categorizing, answering why questions, predicting, sequencing, identifying cause and effect, and role playing.			✔			*	✔	✔	✔
On My Own at Home by Deborah McGraw House and Gloria Nelson. Contains information about real-life topics (e.g., housing, safety, medical information) with discussion questions and ideas for role playing.		✔	✔			*	✔	✔	
On My Own With Language by Betty Stiefel. Contains basic information about real-life situations (e.g., food preparation, travel, jobs) with discussion questions and ideas for role playing.		✔		*		*	✔	✔	
Problem Solving for Teens by Barbara J. Gray. Contains problem solving activities such as making choices, planning actions, checking results, and avoiding problems.						*	✔		

	Process							
	A	M	ORG	O	P	PR	PJ	R	S
RAPP (Resource of Activities for Peer Pragmatics) by Nancy L. McConnell and Carolyn M. Blagden. Consists of practical exercises in such things as using body language, interrupting politely, asking the right questions, and recognizing intonation clues.						✔		✔	
WALC (Workbook of Activities for Language and Cognition) by Kathryn J. Tomlin. Contains activities in the areas of attention and concentration, memory for general information, visual and auditory memory, sequential thought, and reasoning.	✔	✔	✔		✔		✔	✔	

Midwest Publications
P.O. Box 448
Pacific Grove, CA 93950

Basic Thinking Skills by Anita Harnadek.

	A	M	ORG	O	P	PR	PJ	R	S
"Analogies: A-D" Contains exercises for the interpretation and use of analogies.								✔	✔
"Antonyms and Synonyms" Contains exercises for identifying and providing antonyms and synonyms.								✔	✔
"Antonyms, Synonyms, Similarities and Differences" Contains exercises for identifying and providing antonyms, synonyms, similarities, and differences.			✔					✔	✔
"Following Directions A, B" Contains paper and pencil activities for following increasingly complex directions.	✔	✔			✔				
"Miscellaneous, Including Transitivity and Same Person or Not?" Contains activities for perceiving relationships and drawing conclusions.			✔					✔	
"Patterns" Contains exercises for analysis and synthesis of visual patterns.					✔			✔	

	Process							
A	M	ORG	O	P	PR	PJ	R	S

"Think About It"
Contains problem solving exercises requiring deductions and inferences.

						*	✔	

"What Would You Do?" and "True to Life, or Fantasy?"
Contains activities for solving hypothetical everyday problems and determining fact from fantasy.

						✔	✔	

Building Thinking Skills: Books l, 2, 3 Figural, 3 Verbal by Howard and Sandra Black.
Contains exercises for identification of figural and verbal similarities and differences, sequencing, classification, drawing analogies, and deductive reasoning.

		✔	✔	✔			✔	✔

Challenging Codes: Riddles and Jokes by Karen E. Morrell.
Contains exercises for deciphering symbols to formulate riddles and jokes.

✔		✔					✔	✔

Connector Vectors: Books A, B, C by John H. Doolittle.
Contains exercises for analyzing and generating related words and concepts.

						✔	✔	✔

Critical Thinking Activities to Improve Writing Skills by K. Albertus, B. Baker, M. Baker, C. Bannes, G. Dietrich, and E. Korver.

"Arguments"
Contains activities for developing solutions to a given problem.

					*	✔	✔	

"Where-Abouts"
Contains such exercises as map reading and following directions.

			✔		*		✔	

"Descriptive Mysteries"
Contains exercises to facilitate object descriptions.

					*			✔

Inductive Thinking Skills by Anita Harnadek.

"Cause and Effect"
Contains problems designed to differentiate be-

							✔	

tween events that have a cause and effect and those that are simultaneous, coincidental, or somehow related.

"Figure Patterns"
Contains activities for analyzing and determining the relationships between figures.

"Inferences A, B"
Contains activities for drawing reasonable inferences from information about real-life situations and evaluating their appropriateness.

"Open- Ended Problems"
Contains activities designed to stimulate analysis and synthesis of everyday situations and develop alternate strategies for dealing with them.

"Reasoning by Analogy"
Contains activities designed to analyze analogous everyday situations and evaluate their merits.

"Relevant Information"
Contains activities for determining relevancy of a statement to a given problem.

Mind Benders A1-A3, B1-B3, C1-C3 by Anita Harnadek.
Contains exercises for organizing sets of information and reaching logical conclusions through deductive reasoning.

Organizing Thinking by Howard and Sandra Black.
Contains activities for organizing information and illustrating relationships in a visual format.

Syllogisms: Beginning 1, 2, Books A, B, C by Michael Baker.
Contains syllogistic exercises for deductive reasoning.

Thinking About Time: Books 1, 2, 3 by Randy Wiseman.
Contains activities such as sequencing days of the week and months, making up schedules, reading a calendar, and writing dates numerically.

| | | | | Process | | | | |
A	M	ORG	O	P	PR	PJ	R	S
				✔			✔	
						✔	✔	
						✔	✔	
						✔	✔	
							✔	
		✔					✔	
		✔					✔	✔
							✔	
✔	✔	✔						

		Process						
A	M	ORG	O	P	PR	PJ	R	S

Verbal Classifications: Books B, C by Howard and Sandra Black.

Contains exercises for categorizing words by meaning, use, or characteristics.

→ ORG ✔, S ✔

Verbal Sequences: Books A, B, C by Howard and Sandra Black.

Contains exercises for verbal sequencing of words, phrases, and sentences.

→ ORG ✔, S ✔

What Would You Do?: Books A, B by Michael O. Baker.

Contains exercises for analyzing everyday situations, developing solutions, and predicting consequences.

→ PR *, PJ ✔, R ✔

New Readers Press
Division of Laubach Literacy International
P.O. Box 131
Syracuse, NY 13210

Challenger 1-8 by Corea Murphy.

Consists of an eight book program of stimulating adult level material followed by a variety of exercises and activities.

→ M *, ORG *, PJ *, R *, S *

Cliffhangers by Henry Billings.

Contains exercises in which the endings to true stories must be provided, facts must be recalled, and events kept in order.

→ M ✔, ORG ✔, PJ ✔

Everyday Reading and Writing by Frank Laubach, Elizabeth Kirk, and Robert Laubach.

Contains practical everyday activities such as reading signs, maps, and reference books and writing business and personal letters.

→ M *, ORG *, O *, PJ *

Feelings Illustrated.

Consists of black and white photos with captions illustrating the feelings associated with laughing, working, playing, and loving.

→ PR *, PJ *

Feelings, Thoughts and Dreams: Writing and Conversation Starters by Fran Reed.

Contains short, simple readings that stimulate discussion.

→ PR ✔, PJ ✔, R ✔

				Process				
A	M	ORG	O	P	PR	PJ	R	S

Filling Out Forms by Wendy Stein.

Contains exercises for filling out applications and forms.

A	M	ORG	O	P	PR	PJ	R	S
	*	*						

News for You.

Consists of four page weekly newspaper with high interest, large print, adult level material at a fourth to sixth grade reading level.

A	M	ORG	O	P	PR	PJ	R	S
	*					*	*	*

Practice in Survival Reading

Consists of materials such as newspaper items, maps, and product labels followed by factual and interpretive questions.

A	M	ORG	O	P	PR	PJ	R	S
	*	*	✔	*			✔	

Book 2—"Signs around Town" by Calvin Greatsinger.
Book 3—"Label Talk" by Calvin Greatsinger.
Book 4—"Read the Instructions First" by Calvin Greatsinger.
Book 5—"Your Daily Paper" by Wendy Stein.
Book 6—"It's on the Map" by Patricia Waelder.
Book 7—"Let's Look It Up" by Patricia Waelder.
Book 8—"Caution: Fine Print Ahead" by Patricia Waelder.

You are Here: A Guide to Everyday Maps, Plans and Diagrams by Stephen A. Martin.

Contains illustrated, easy-to-follow instructions for reading maps, plans, and diagrams covering such topics as city, road, and weather maps, floor plans, and transit maps.

A	M	ORG	O	P	PR	PJ	R	S
			✔					

Pro-Ed
8700 Shoal Creek
Austin, TX 78758-6897

Auditory Rehabilitation: Memory-Language-Comprehension by Rex Pater and Karlene Stefanakos.

Contains exercises that progress from the retrieval of one fact from a 7- to 10-word oral presentation to the retrieval of five facts and the drawing of two inferential conclusions from a 5- to 9-sentence oral presentation.

A	M	ORG	O	P	PR	PJ	R	S
	✔						✔	

Cognitive Reorganization: A Stimulus Handbook by Elizabeth J. Bressler and Sharon M. Holloran.

A	M	ORG	O	P	PR	PJ	R	S
	✔	✔	✔			✔	✔	✔

	Process								
	A	M	ORG	O	P	PR	PJ	R	S

Contains activities increasing in order of difficulty in the areas of orientation and memory, simple relationships and associations, simple problem solving, abstract reasoning, functional problem solving, independent information management, and functional activities of daily living.

Language Rehabilitation by James T. Martinoff, Rosemary Martinoff, and Virginia Stokke.

"Auditory Comprehension"
Contains exercises for following directions and auditory comprehension and reasoning tasks at the word, sentence, and paragraph level.

A	M	ORG	O	P	PR	PJ	R	S
✔	✔	✔					✔	

"Reading"
Contains exercises for single words, sentence, and paragraph material.

A	M	ORG	O	P	PR	PJ	R	S
							✔	✔

"Verbal Expression"
Contains exercises for sequencing words into sentences and sentences into paragraphs, explaining idioms, and formulating opinions.

A	M	ORG	O	P	PR	PJ	R	S
*	*	✔				✔	✔	✔

"Written Expression"
Contains exercises such as categorizing, sequencing words into sentences, changing questions to statements, and identifying words within a block of letters.

A	M	ORG	O	P	PR	PJ	R	S
		✔		✔	✔	✔		✔

Lessons for the Right Brain by Kathleen Anderson and Pamela Crowe Miller.

"Memory Workbook"
Contains exercises for recall of daily activities, seasons, months of the year, shapes, words, and pictures.

A	M	ORG	O	P	PR	PJ	R	S
	✔	✔	✔				*	

"Reading and Writing Workbook"
Contains functional reading and writing activities.

A	M	ORG	O	P	PR	PJ	R	S
			✔	✔				✔

"Self Perception/Organizing Functional Information Workbook"
Contains exercises for body part recognition, right and left discrimination, emotions, humor, and personal problem solving.

A	M	ORG	O	P	PR	PJ	R	S
		✔	✔		✔	✔	✔	

				Process					
	A	M	ORG	O	P	PR	PJ	R	S
"Thought Organization Workbook" Contains letter and word puzzles and exercises for sequencing shapes, numbers, events, words, and sentences.			✔	✔				✔	✔
"Visual Perception and Attention Workbook" Contains exercises for visual discrimination, spatial organization, visual scanning, and clock imagery.	✔			✔	✔				
Let's Organize Today by Roberta DePompei and Jean Blosser. Contains suggestions, in a calendar format, of over 375 language based daily activities to facilitate changes in language skills and increase communicative interactions.		✔	✔	✔		✔	✔	✔	✔
PALS: Pragmatic Activities in Language and Speech by Betty X. Davis. Contains exercises in non-verbal communication, active listening, remembering, speaking, and reading in areas such as telephoning, job interviewing, and filling in forms and applications.		✔				✔			✔
Photo Sequence Cards: Complete Program. Contains sets of photographs in the areas of occupations, recreation, and daily living activities. There are 10 different concepts in each set and each concept is illustrated by 4 photos for sequencing.				✔					
Rebuilding Language: Auditory Comprehension, Word Retrieval, Syntax by Mary Rambow and Terry L. Latham. Contains exercises arranged in a hierarchy of complexity in the areas of auditory comprehension (e.g., following commands, answering "wh" questions), word retrieval (e.g., generating a story, engaging in conversation), and syntax (e.g., sequencing sentences, generating solutions to problems).		✔	*			*	*		
The Psychological Corporation 555 Academic Court San Antonio, TX 78204-2498									
Let's Talk: Developing Prosocial Communication Skills by Elisabeth H. Wiig.						✔	✔		

					Process				
A	*M*	*ORG*	*O*	*P*	*PR*	*PJ*	*R*	*S*

Contains card games emphasizing functional communication skills in such situations as shopping and getting around town and with such intents as sharing feelings and asking for favors.

Let's Talk: Intermediate Level by Elisabeth H. Wiig.

Contains situation and activity cards in the following areas: signs, labels, and warnings; places and directions; invitations and suggestions; favors and assistance; and choices.

Words, Expressions and Contexts: A Figurative Language Program by Elisabeth Wiig.

Contains activity and situation cards to teach strategies for understanding figurative uses of words, concepts, and metaphors.

Quercus
Simon & Schuster School Group
4343 Equity Drive
P.O. Box 26499
Columbus, OH 43216

Consumer Skills for Living on Your Own by Beverly Keller.

Contains information for budget planning and decision making skills in such budget categories as savings, housing, transportation, and entertainment. An activity book is available with exercises to reinforce these skills.

Get That Job by Carol Lindsay and Corinn Scott.

Contains information focusing on applying for a social security card, completing job applications, and interviewing.

Owning A Car by Patrick Kelley.

Contains diagrams and narratives explaining car operation, maintenance, insurance, and handling emergencies.

Paying with Cash by Marjorie Kelley.

Contains activities for counting money, recognizing coins and bills, making exact change, and counting change for purchases.

Item	*A*	*M*	*ORG*	*O*	*P*	*PR*	*PJ*	*R*	*S*
Let's Talk: Intermediate Level						✔	✔		
Words, Expressions and Contexts						✔	✔	✔	
Consumer Skills for Living on Your Own			✔				✔		
Get That Job			∗			∗			
Owning A Car						∗	∗		
Paying with Cash		∗	∗				∗		

					Process				
	A	M	ORG	O	P	PR	PJ	R	S
Paying with Promises by Marjorie Kelley.						*	*		
The Telephone Book Can Help You by Yehudit Goldfarb.		*			*		*		
The Way to Work by Marjorie Kelley.						*	*		
Corrective Reading Comprehension: Concept Applications by Siegfried Engelmann et al.	✔	✔						✔	
The Curious Reader: Increasing Comprehension and Vocabulary Skills: Book 1–7 by Bernice H. Baumer.	*	✔					*		✔
"Cleaning Up Your Act"	*					✔	✔	✔	

Paying with Promises by Marjorie Kelley.

   Contains information about the advantages and disadvantages of using money orders, lay away plans, checks, coupons, mail order, credit cards, and taking out loans.

The Telephone Book Can Help You by Yehudit Goldfarb.

   Contains information about finding numbers for people, places, and services in the white and yellow pages, interpreting abbreviations for names and addresses, and finding and using emergency numbers.

The Way to Work by Marjorie Kelley.

   Contains information and exercises focusing on the way to work and how to apply problem-solving techniques to various jobs.

Science Research Associates, Inc. (SRA)
155 N. Wacker Drive
Chicago, IL 60606

Corrective Reading Comprehension: Concept Applications by Siegfried Engelmann et al.

   Contains exercises such as analyzing advertisements and editorials, evaluating sources of information, and organizing information for retention and reporting.

The Curious Reader: Increasing Comprehension and Vocabulary Skills: Book 1–7 by Bernice H. Baumer.

   Contains exercises focusing on such areas as finding the main idea, recalling details, sequencing, and outlining.

Learning Through Reading by Noel E. Bowling, Iva Dean Cook, and Diana Salyers.

   (An audiotape is available for each of the following books.)

   "Cleaning Up Your Act"
   Contains activities focusing on such topics as cleanliness, benefits of exercise, choosing clothes, and maintaining your wardrobe.

			Process						
	A	*M*	*ORG*	*O*	*P*	*PR*	*PJ*	*R*	*S*
"A Night on the Town" Contains activities focusing on such topics as thinking before acting, gathering facts, anticipating costs, resolving problems, and taking risks.		*	✔			✔	✔	✔	
"The Payoff" Contains activities focusing on such topics as being on time to work, working with co-workers, communication with customers, and accepting responsibility.		*		✔		✔			
"Serious Business" Contains activities focusing on such topics as locating job opportunities, recognizing job qualifications, applying for a job, and preparing for an interview.		*				✔	✔		
"The Wallet War" Contains activities focusing on such topics as shopping for bargains, comparing prices, checking ingredients, and saving time.		*	✔			✔	✔		
Math for Independence by Kathy Jungjohann and Becky Roth Schenck. Contains activities focusing on such areas as using checking and savings accounts, basic units of time, making change, and reading temperatures. "How to Manage Your Money" "How to Understand and Manage Your Time" "How to Use Bank Accounts" "How to Use Measurements"			✔	✔			✔		
Reading For Independence by Kathy Jungjohann and Becky Roth Schenck. "How to Follow Directions" Contains activities focusing on recognizing and following common directions such as traffic signs, recipes, first aid guides, and washing instructions.		*	✔						
"How to Use Maps and Directories" Contains exercises focusing on how to use maps to plan trips and find locations.				✔	✔				

				Process					
	A	M	ORG	O	P	PR	PJ	R	S
"How to Use the Classified Ads" Contains exercises focusing on finding bargains, jobs, and services, and differentiating between terms such as for sale and on sale.			✔		✔				
"How to Use the Newspaper" Contains activities focusing on making informed and independent decisions about purchasing, safety, apartment living, and the news.	✱		✔	✱	✔				
"How to Use Schedules" Contains activities focusing on using timetables for buses, movies, and classes.				✔	✔				
"How to Use the Telephone Book" Contains activities focusing on finding addresses and phone numbers in the white and yellow pages.			✔		✔				
Writing for Independence by Kathy Jungjohann and Becky Roth Schenck. Contains activities focusing on taking phone messages, completing job applications, writing resumes, and filling in tax forms. "How to Complete Job Applications and Resumes" "How to Manage Your Personal Affairs" "How to Write Letters and Messages"	✔	✔							
Real-Life English: Books 1–4 by Julia Jolly and Lynne Robinson. Contains exercises to facilitate appropriate conversation and self-monitoring in everyday situations.						✔			
"Consumer Issues" Contains exercises with real-life scenarios such as resolving consumer complaints, using community resources, and filling out forms.						✱	✱	✱	
"Everyday People" Contains exercises focusing on real-life situations such as landlord problems and elderly care.						✱	✱	✱	

Steck-Vaugh
P.O. Box 26015
Austin, TX 78755

Real-Life Reading by Annie DeCaprio.

| | Process | | | | | | | |
	A	M	ORG	O	P	PR	PJ	R	S

Vocabulary Connections: Level F-H by Barbara Coulter, Catherine Hatala, and Carole Arnold (program consultants).

Contains reading selections followed by such exercises as analogies, using context, word puzzles, and developing dictionary skills.

Therapy Skill Builders
3830 E. Bellevue
P.O. Box 42050-C90
Tucson, AZ 85733

Cognitive Rehabilitation: Group Games and Activities by Joan P. Toglia and Kathleen M. Golisz.

Consists of group table-top games that can be played in such formats as moving around a board and answering questions or answering questions quickly within a competitive game.

Essential Life Skill Series by Carolyn Morton Starkey and Norgina Wright Penn.

Contains five books with a variety of activities in the following areas: reading labels, directions and newspapers; reading signs, directories, schedules, maps, charts, and utility bills; basic writing skills, letters, and consumer complaints; reading ads, reference materials, and legal documents; and getting a job and filling out forms.

Focus on Function: Retraining for the Communicatively Impaired Client by Shelly E. Hahn and Evelyn Klein.

Consists of practical activities in the five skill areas of verbal, phone, reading, writing, and numerical functions.

Winterberry City: Map Games and Activities for Language and Problem Solving by Sharon Foley Eastvold.

Consists of map games and activities designed to improve every day skills such as decoding a bus schedule and looking up information in the telephone directory.

Title	A	M	ORG	O	P	PR	PJ	R	S
Vocabulary Connections: Level F-H		*						✔	✔
Cognitive Rehabilitation: Group Games and Activities		✔		✔		✔			
Essential Life Skill Series		*	✔	✔	✔				✔
Focus on Function			✔			✔	✔	✔	✔
Winterberry City: Map Games and Activities			✔	✔	✔		✔		

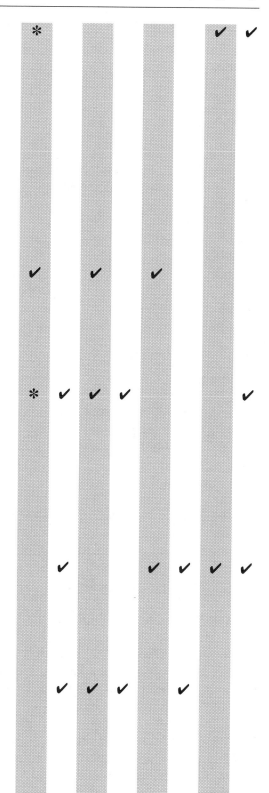

	Process								
	A	M	ORG	O	P	PR	PJ	R	S

Thinking Publications
1731 Westgate Road
P.O. Box 163
Eau Claire, WI 54702-0163

ALP—Active Listening Program by Carrie van der Laan. — A ✔, M ✔

Contains materials that progress from simple to complex listening activities that simulate classroom lectures, news presentations, job situations, and other daily activities.

Daily Communication: Strategies for the Language Disordered Adolescent by Linda Schwartz and Nancy McKinley. — PR ✔, PJ ✔, R ✔

Contains activities in the areas of problem solving, listening, conversational skills, question asking, nonverbal communication, study skills, and survival language.

Scripting: Social Communication for Adolescents by Patty Mayo and Patti Waldo. — PR ✔

Consists of scripts addressing 53 social communication skills such as getting to the point, making an apology, and expressing humor. Appropriate and inappropriate examples of each skill are provided to promote discussion.

Referential Communication (Part Two) by Linda Schwartz and Nancy McKinley. — A ✔, M ✔, P ✔, PR ✔

Contains pattern cards and die-cut forms to be used for barrier activities requiring the sending and receiving of clear and precise messages.

Social Skill Strategies (Books A, B) by Nancy Gajewski and Patty Mayo. — PR ✔, PJ ✔

Contain structured activities and discussion topics to teach social skills such as introducing people, convincing others, expressing feelings, and giving and accepting constructive criticism.

Warm-up Exercises: Calisthenics for the Brain (Books 1, 2) by Rita Kisner and Brooke Knowles. — A ✔, M ✔, P ✔, PR ✔, S ✔

Contain short exercises in areas such as auditory perception and memory, general questions, and classification.

	A	M	ORG	O	P	PR	PJ	R	S
Process									

Wayne State University Press
5959 Woodward Avenue
Detroit, MI 48202

Workbook for Aphasia (Revised Edition) by Susan Howell Brubaker.
   Contains a variety of exercises targeting such areas as word usage, concrete and abstract reasoning, and personal experiences.

Workbook for Cognitive Skills by Susan Howell Brubaker.
   Contains a variety of exercises such as visual recognition, logic puzzles, map reading, and multiple meanings.

Workbook for Language Skills: Exercises for Written and Verbal Expression by Susan Howell Brubaker.
   Contains a variety of exercises targeting such areas as figurative language, general knowledge, and word recall.

Workbook for Reasoning Skills: Exercises for Cognitive Facilitation by Susan Howell Brubaker.
   Contains a variety of exercises targeting the areas of drawing conclusions, problem solving, following directions, visual/logical sequencing, humor, and numbers/symbols.

United Education Services, Inc.
P.O. Box 605
East Aurora, NY 14052

Language for Living by Jean R. Neils, Bradford E. Weisiger, and Amy R. Martin.
   Consists of eight workbooks addressing auditory/verbal, reading/writing, working with numbers, and home activities using topics such as games, sports, shopping, home, and auto.

Visiting Nurse Service
1200 McArthur Drive
Akron, OH 44320

Putting the Pieces Together by Kathryn M. Kilpatrick.

Title	A	M	ORG	O	P	PR	PJ	R	S
Workbook for Aphasia (Revised Edition)		✔			✔		✔	✔	✔
Workbook for Cognitive Skills		✔	✔	✔				✔	✔
Workbook for Language Skills								✔	✔
Workbook for Reasoning Skills		✔					✔	✔	
Language for Living	✔	✔	✔						✔
Putting the Pieces Together		✔			✔		✔		

				Process					
	A	M	ORG	O	P	PR	PJ	R	S
Contains a variety of exercises targeting the areas of visual-spatial reasoning, verbal reasoning, and numerical reasoning.									

Therapy Guide for Language and Speech Disorders

	A	M	ORG	O	P	PR	PJ	R	S
Volume 1: *A Selection of Stimulus Materials* by Kathryn M. Kilpatrick, Cynthia Jones, and Janis Reller. Contains a variety of exercises such as multiple meanings, identifying situations, and categorization.	✔	✱	✔				✔	✔	✔
Volume 1: *Spanish Version* by Ingrid Bahler and Katherine Gye Kenyest Gatto. Contains above materials in Spanish.	✔	✱	✔				✔	✔	✔
Volume 2: *Advanced Stimulus Materials* by Kathryn M. Kilpatrick. Contains a variety of exercises targeting such areas as general knowledge, thought organization, and daily needs.			✔			✱	✔	✔	✔
Volume 5: *Reading Comprehension Materials* by Kathryn M. Kilpatrick. Contains stimulus materials of increasing length, followed by questions.		✱							
Working with Words by Kathryn M. Kilpatrick. Contains a variety of puzzles and word games.		✔			✔				✔

Commercially Available Computer Programs

KEY

Process

A   = Attention
M   = Memory
ORG = Organization
O   = Orientation
P   = Perception
PR   = Pragmatics
PJ   = Problem Solving/Judgment
R   = Reasoning
S   = Semantics

| | *Process* | | | | | | | |
	A	M	ORG	O	P	PR	PJ	R	S
Blaca P.O. Box 3186 Kent, OH 44240 *Reading the Newspaper: Sports and World/National News* by Robert S. Pierce. Consists of 110 short (4–6 lines) and long (10–12 lines) newspaper articles followed by questions.		✔							✔
Cambridge Development Laboratory, Inc. 214 Third Avenue Waltham, MA 02154 *Map Skills* by Weekly Reader. Consists of five maps with 20 trips each that teach map reading.				✔					
Mind Castle I & II by MCE. Consists of an adventure game that requires reasoning skills, critical reading, and spatial orientation.						✔		✔ ✔	

				Process				
A	M	ORG	O	P	PR	PJ	R	S

Money Management by Marshware.

Consists of activities that require planning and controlling personal finances including dealing with credit cards, loans, mortgage, and retirement income.

| | | ✔ | | | | | ✔ | |

Think Quick by The Learning Company.

Consists of an interactive adventure game that requires interpreting maps, deciphering codes, designing strategies, managing resources, and making decisions quickly.

| | | | ✔ | | | ✔ | ✔ | |

Where in Europe Is Carmen Sandiego? by Broderbund.

Consists of a game that requires deductive reasoning and reference and research skills.

| | | ✔ | | | | ✔ | ✔ | |

Where in the U.S.A. Is Carmen Sandiego? by Broderbund.

Consists of a game that helps develop language and problem solving skills.

| | | ✔ | | | | ✔ | ✔ | |

Where in the World Is Carmen Sandiego? by Broderbund.

Consists of a game that requires solving clues to reach the goal; emphasizes taking notes and using reference sources.

| | | ✔ | | | | ✔ | ✔ | |

Where in Time Is Carmen Sandiego? by Broderbund.

Consists of a game that requires solving clues to reach the goal.

| | | ✔ | | | | ✔ | ✔ | |

Communication Skill Builders
3830 E. Bellevue
P.O. Box 42050-AC
Tucson, AZ 85733

Ace Reporter by Mindplay.

Consists of activities that require reading for detail and main ideas.

| | ✔ | ✔ | | | | | | |

Idioms in America by Carol Esterreicher.

Consists of activities that require creating an original sentence using idioms.

| | | | | | | | ✔ | |

Wizard of Words by Anita Neely and Tim Aaronson.

| | | ✔ | | | | | ✔ | |

	Process							
A	*M*	*ORG*	*O*	*P*	*PR*	*PJ*	*R*	*S*

Consists of games that require unscrambling words, creative crossword puzzles, and finding mystery words.

The Continental Press, Inc.
520 E. Bainbridge St.
Elizabeth, PA 17022

Reading for Comprehension Software.
Consists of high-interest narratives with questions focusing on main ideas and details, inferences, sequences, cause and effect, and fact and opinion; contains a built-in reward game.

A	M	ORG	O	P	PR	PJ	R	S
✔	✔						✔	✔

EBSCO Curriculum Materials
Division of EBSCO Industries, Inc.
Box 11542
Birmingham, AL 35201

Word Works 1, 2, & 3.
Consists of three programs that create 20 different worksheets using your words and definitions; activities include scrambled words, word search, missing letters, and crossword puzzles.

A	M	ORG	O	P	PR	PJ	R	S
		✔						✔

Word Works: Data Disks for Deductive Reasoning.
Contains exercises for word analogies and classification that are used in conjunction with *Word Works 1, 2 & 3.*

A	M	ORG	O	P	PR	PJ	R	S
		✔					✔	✔

Gamco Industries, Inc.
P.O. Box 1862S6
Big Springs, TX 79721-1862

Reading and Thinking II & IV.
Consists of reading passages followed by questions that require making inferences.

A	M	ORG	O	P	PR	PJ	R	S
							✔	

Reading for Information.
Consists of activities such as: finding chapters and articles by topic, alphabetically, and numerically; finding names in a telephone directory; and typing the corresponding telephone numbers.

A	M	ORG	O	P	PR	PJ	R	S
			✔	✔				

	Process								
	A	M	ORG	O	P	PR	PJ	R	S
Word Search Puzzles. Consists of a program in which the clinician can select the list to use for the word search puzzle, the number of words to be hidden, the number of rows and columns in the puzzle, and the direction in which the words will appear (vertical, horizontal, forward, backward, and/or diagonal).					✔				
Hartley Courseware Inc. Box 419 Dimondale, MI 48821									
Analogies Advanced. Consists of a program which provides advanced work in analogies.								✔	✔
Analogies College Bound. Consists of an advanced analogies program similar to the analogy questions on college entrance tests.								✔	✔
Analogies Tutorial. Consists of a tutorial which teaches identifying and solving analogies.								✔	✔
Cognitive Rehabilitation. Consists of five separate programs organized from simple to complex and targets such areas as categorization, sequencing, association, and memory; also includes an authoring program for expanding or individualizing activities from the core area.	✔	✔						✔	✔
Drawing Conclusions and Problem Solving. Consists of exercises in inferential reasoning and problem solving.							✔	✔	
Fact or Opinion. Consists of a program designed to distinguish facts and opinions.								✔	
Memory Match. Consists of a concentration game which contains 25 lessons including such categories as opposites, digit and number words, rhyming words, and homonyms.	✔	✔							

	Process								
	A	M	ORG	O	P	PR	PJ	R	S
Multiple Meanings. Consists of exercises for working on a number of different meanings for the same word.								✔	✔
Using a Calendar. Consists of exercises in reading and interpreting a calendar.				✔					

Imaginart Communication Products
307 Arizona St.
Bisbee, AZ 85603

	A	M	ORG	O	P	PR	PJ	R	S
Cognitive Software: Visual Tasks by Richard Katz. Consists of a series of 11 programs with activities involving attention, reaction time, visual field, visual scanning, visual discrimination, and memory skills.	✔	✔			✔				
Understanding Sentences I & II by Richard Katz. Consists of activities to identify the absurd word in a sentence and to interpret the meaning of metaphors.								✔	✔

Laureate Learning Systems, Inc.
110 East Spring St.
Winooski, VT 05404

	A	M	ORG	O	P	PR	PJ	R	S
Bozons' Quest by Bernard J. Fox and Mary Sweig Wilson. Consists of a game that requires memory, planning, and decision-making, and reinforces right-left discrimination skills.		✔		✔			✔	✔	
Concentrate: On Words and Concepts I, II & III by Mary Sweig Wilson and Bernard J. Fox. Consists of games (based on the classic card game, Concentration) in which the players try to find a match based on vocabulary, categorization, word identification by function, or word association.	✔	✔							✔
First Categories by Mary Sweig Wilson and Bernard J. Fox. Consists of 60 nouns in 6 categories to train categorization by inclusion or exclusion with or without cuing.				✔					✔
Twenty Categories by Mary Sweig Wilson and Bernard J. Fox.				✔					✔

Consists of 300 nouns and 20 categories with questions which train categorization concepts in three ways—Inclusion Category to Noun, Inclusion Noun to Category, and Exclusion Category to Noun.

Words and Concepts I, II & III by Mary Sweig Wilson.

Consists of three programs each containing a core vocabulary of 40 nouns and includes such activities as categorization, word association, and concepts of same and different.

Learning Well
CS 9001, Dept. 590
Roslyn Heights, NY 11577-9001

Drawing Conclusions/Chief of Detectives.

Consists of high interest reading selections to be analyzed for hidden meanings.

Fact or Opinion/Smart Shopper.

Consists of a realistic shopping excursion that helps develop critical reading skills.

Following Directions/Behind the Wheel.

Consists of an automobile race that requires reading comprehension, thinking, and memory skills.

Jumbles.
Consists of exercises for unscrambling words.

Moptown Hotel.

Consists of activities that develop the use of analogies, sequences, and hypotheses.

Sequence/What Comes First.

Consists of activities that require unscrambling words, sentences, and paragraphs.

Wordsearch.

Consists of exercises that involve searching for words hidden vertically, diagonally, upside down, or backwards.

Item	A	M	ORG	O	P	PR	PJ	R	S
Words and Concepts I, II & III			✔					✔	✔
Drawing Conclusions/Chief of Detectives								✔	
Fact or Opinion/Smart Shopper						✔		✔	
Following Directions/Behind the Wheel	✔			✔				✔	
Jumbles			✔						
Moptown Hotel			✔					✔	
Sequence/What Comes First			✔						
Wordsearch					✔				

	Process	A	M	ORG	O	P	PR	PJ	R	S

Midwest Publications
P.O. Box 448
Pacific Grove, CA 93950

Hangtown by John Doolittle, program by E. Thornton.
   Consists of three games (Hangtown, Farmtown, and Pirate Island) that require using familiar objects in unfamiliar ways and mapping out the environment so as to mentally manipulate information, ideas, and objects.

Process: ORG, O, PJ, R

Math Mind Benders by Anita Harnadek, program by E. Thornton.
   Consists of games that require solving puzzles using mathematical/verbal deductive reasoning.

Process: R

Mind Benders by Anita Harnadek, program by B. Boening.
   Consists of games that require solving a word problem by deducing information from a clue.

Process: M, R

Roller Dog by Michael Baker, program by E. Thornton.
   Contains games which require spatial rotation/figural reasoning skills and reinforce critical thinking skills.

Process: P, R

What's My Logic by Michael Baker, program by E. Thornton, T. Valleau, and J. Hampton.

   "What's My Logic?—Figural"
   Contains 20 different mazes that require the player to use inductive and deductive reasoning to determine the logical rule for each game.

Process: R

   "What's My Logic?—Figural/Verbal"
   Contains 20 different mazes each of which requires players to convert words to images (or vice versa) as they create a logical path to the goal.

Process: R, S

Milliken Publishing Co.
1100 Research Blvd.
P.O. Box 21579
St. Louis, MO 63132-0579

	A	M	ORG	O	P	PR	PJ	R	S
Process									

Problem Solving.

Consists of problems that require planning, predicting, experimenting, testing, and analyzing results.

Parrot Software
P.O. Box 1139
State College, PA 16804-1139

Aphasia X: Orientation for Aphasia and Cognitive Disorders: Mastering Personal Information by Alan Gallaher and Frederick F. Weiner.

Consists of activities to practice copying, revisualization, and recall of orienting information.

Cognitive Disorders 1: Category Naming and Completion by Lorrie Houston Dillon and Frederick F. Weiner.

Consists of activities that require determining the category of a short list of words and then adding a word to that list.

Cognitive Disorders 2: Category Discrimination and Reasoning by Lorrie Houston Dillon and Frederick F. Weiner.

Consists of problems that require determining which word in the list does not belong, the reason it does not belong, and an appropriate word to replace the incorrect one.

Cognitive Disorders 3: Attention/Perception by Lorrie Houston Dillon and Frederick F. Weiner.

Consists of activities that require matching geometric, alphabetic, or numeric shapes.

Cognitive Disorders 4: Memory for Pictures by Alice Kamin, Merle Joblin, and Frederick F. Weiner.

Consists of activities that require recall of pictures; incorporates distraction in the form of visual and auditory interference.

Cognitive Disorders 5: Cognitive Retraining with Print Shop Pictures by Frederick F. Weiner.

Consists of an authoring program that allows the user to create lessons using pictures on the picture disk or the print shop program.

Title	A	M	ORG	O	P	PR	PJ	R	S
Problem Solving							✔	✔	
Aphasia X	✔			✔					
Cognitive Disorders 1			✔						✔
Cognitive Disorders 2			✔					✔	✔
Cognitive Disorders 3	✔				✔				
Cognitive Disorders 4	✔	✔							
Cognitive Disorders 5	Flexible: Depends on Program Developed								

	Process								
	A	M	ORG	O	P	PR	PJ	R	S
Cognitive Disorders 6: Verbal Analogies by Frederick F. Weiner and Matthew J. Weiner. Consists of analogy exercises.								✔	
Cognitive Disorders 7: Word Order in Sentences by Matthew J. Weiner and Frederick F. Weiner. Consists of activities that require unscrambling words to form sentences.			✔						
Cognitive Disorders 8: Inferential Naming for Cognitive Language Disorders by Lorrie Houston Dillon and Frederick F. Weiner. Consists of activities that require generating a word from its semantic features such as category, function, location and size, shape, or color.			✔					✔	✔
Cognitive Disorders 9: Sorting by Category by Frederick F. Weiner. Consists of activities that require sorting of words into categories.			✔						✔
Cognitive Disorders 10: Categories: Completion from Partial Information by Frederick F. Weiner. Consists of activities that require generating a word from part of the word and its category.			✔						✔
Cognitive Disorders 11: Semantic Development Using Code Breaking Strategies by Matt Weiner. Consists of activities that require determining an unknown sentence using an alphanumeric code.			✔		✔			✔	
Hierarchical Attention Training by Lorrie Houston Dillon and Frederick F. Weiner. Consists of activities for focused alternating, and divided attention.	✔								

A.W. Peller and Associates, Inc.
Educational Materials
210 Sixth Ave.
P.O. Box 106
Hawthorne, NJ 07507

Brain Booster. Consists of activities designed to increase reasoning by visual analogy.								✔	

		Process							
	A	M	ORG	O	P	PR	PJ	R	S
Cause and Effect. Consists of activities that require inductive and deductive reasoning.								✔	
Mind over Matter. Consists of 185 word puzzles that use symbols and graphics to facilitate creative and deductive thinking.								✔	
Perplexing Puzzles. Consists of problems designed to develop logical reasoning and critical reading and questioning.							✔	✔	
Probability through Problem Solving. Consists of activities that require solving probability problems.							✔		
Reasoning—The Logical Process. Consists of problems and puzzles designed to develop inductive and deductive reasoning, hypothesis testing, drawing conclusions, and using probability analysis.							✔	✔	
The 4th R—Reasoning. Consists of an interactive introduction to logic that teaches analysis, reasoning, and questioning through imaginative problems and puzzles.								✔	
What's My Logic. Consists of a game that requires inductive and deductive reasoning to learn the concepts of negation, conjunction, inclusion, and exclusion.								✔	

Psychological Corporation
Harcourt Brace Jovanovich Inc.
555 Academic Court
San Antonio, TX 78204-2498

	A	M	ORG	O	P	PR	PJ	R	S
THINKable by IBM. Consists of a program that can be used to construct activities in the areas of visual attention, visual discrimination, visual memory, and visual sequential memory.	✔	✔			✔				

| | Process | | | | | | | |
	A	M	ORG	O	P	PR	PJ	R	S
Psychological Software Services, Inc. 6555 Carrollton Ave. Indianapolis, IN 46220									
Conceptor by Mentor Learning Systems, Inc. Consists of a game that requires perception, classification, and categorization.				✔	✔				
Conceptual by Odie L. Bracy. Consists of computer programs designed to enhance skills involved in relationships, comparisons, and number concepts.				✔					✔
Foundations I by Odie L. Bracy. Consists of computer programs designed to rebuild attention, attention shifting, initiation/inhibition skills, capacity to discriminate, and capacity to respond differentially in both the visual and auditory input modalities.	✔				✔				
Foundations II by Odie L. Bracy. Consists of higher level exercises in the areas of attention, capacity, and vigilance such as visual tracking and scanning.	✔				✔				
Memory I by Odie L. Bracy. Consists of verbal and nonverbal memory exercises via input through visual and auditory mechanisms.		✔							
Memory II by Odie L. Bracy. Consists of verbal and nonverbal memory exercises which also work on encoding, categorizing, and organizing skills.		✔	✔						
Problem Solving by Odie L. Bracy. Consists of tasks such as mazes, cryptograms, and number puzzles requiring logic, reasoning, and strategy development skills.							✔	✔	
Smart Shaper by John Olsen. Consists of basic low level exercises in matching, shape recognition, concepts of same and different, and counting.				✔	✔				

	A	M	ORG	O	P	PR	PJ	R	S
Smart Shaper II by John Olsen. Consists of high level exercises on basic discrimination, matching, and counting.			✔		✔				
Soft Tools '84 by Odie L. Bracy. Consists of a variety of programs including "City Map" (planning a route of travel), "Timesense" (active orientation to time), and "Stars" (counting items as they are added).	✔	✔		✔	✔			✔	
Soft Tools '85 by Odie L. Bracy. Consists of a variety of programs including "Alphabetizing," "Dot-to-Dot," "Scrambled Words," and "Sequenced Memory."		✔	✔		✔				
Soft Tools '86 by Odie L. Bracy. Consists of a variety of programs including "Delayed Memory," "Logic Master" (Mastermind), "Spots" (spatial memory), and "Visual Search."		✔	✔		✔		✔	✔	
Soft Tools '88 by Odie L. Bracy. Consists of a variety of programs including "Alphabit" (visual closure and integration), "Radar" (part/whole analysis, synthesis, and closure), and "Recognize" (attention, perception, and visual discrimination).	✔	✔			✔				
Soft Tools '89 by Odie L. Bracy. Consists of a variety of programs including "Lost" (spatial orientation, mapping, and problem solving), "Reversals" (visual problem solving, prediction, and planning), and "Easy Street" (immediate and delayed recall).		✔		✔	✔		✔	✔	
Visuospatial I by Odie L. Bracy. Consists of computer programs such as mazes, paddleball, and line orientation designed to improve visuoperception and visuomotor integration skills.					✔				
Visuospatial II by Odie L. Bracy. Consists of more complex exercises in the areas of visuoperception and visuomotor integration such as figure/ground and spatial perception.					✔				

				Process				
A	*M*	*ORG*	*O*	*P*	*PR*	*PJ*	*R*	*S*

Queue
338 Commerce Drive
Fairfield, CT 06430

Analytical Reading Skills: B and C.
   Consists of reading comprehension exercises that address the areas of setting (e.g., true to life, historic), plot, characterization, tone (e.g., serious/humorous, sarcastic), and details (e.g., those which describe, persuade, explain, support).
   [P: *, R: ✔]

Drawing Conclusions: Levels D and E.
   Consists of reading comprehension exercises with questions requiring drawing conclusions.
   [R: ✔]

Evaluative Thinking Skills.
   Consists of exercises on: differentiating facts, probabilities, and opinions; determining the author's purpose and point of view; and putting it all together.
   [R: ✔]

Finding the Sequence: Levels D and E.
   Consists of reading comprehension exercises that focus on sequencing.
   [O: ✔]

Finding Cause and Effect: Levels D and E.
   Consists of exercises that require matching a cause with its effect.
   [R: ✔]

Formal Logic I, II, and III.
   Consists of activities that include deductive and inductive inferences, premises and conclusions, truth versus validity, and syllogisms.
   [PJ: ✔, R: ✔]

Getting the Main Idea: Levels D and E.
   Consists of reading comprehension exercises with multiple-choice questions that focus on specific details and require choosing appropriate titles.
   [R: ✔]

Inferential Thinking Skills.
   Consists of lessons on identifying the main idea, judging the adequacy of information, citing evidence, drawing conclusions, and predicting outcomes.
   [O: ✔, PJ: ✔, R: ✔]

Intellectual Decathlon.
   Consists of ten games requiring memory and logic.
   [A: ✔, PJ: ✔, R: ✔]

				Process				
A	M	ORG	O	P	PR	PJ	R	S

Item	A	M	ORG	O	P	PR	PJ	R	S
Literal Reading Skills. Consists of lessons on context, word meaning, sequence, and remembering details.		✔	✔						✔
Making Inferences (RFC): Levels D and E. Consists of reading comprehension exercises that require choosing the most appropriate endings for sentences.								✔	
Memory Builder: Concentration. Consists of a concentration game with words and letters.	✔	✔							
Moon Master. Consists of missing word analogies, true/false analogies, multiple meaning phrases, and multiple meaning riddles.								✔	✔
Noting Details: Levels D and E. Consists of reading comprehension exercises with questions that focus on specific details.				✔					
Predicting Outcomes: Levels D and E. Consists of reading comprehension exercises that require predicting possible outcomes.								✔	
Quick Scramble. Consists of a word game requiring problem solving and vocabulary skills.							✔	✔	✔
Reading Comprehension Series II. Consists of five disks with reading comprehension exercises in each of the following areas: extracting the main idea; recognizing details; sequential order; forming inferences; and fact and opinion.				✔				✔	
Reading and Thinking: II, III and IV. Consists of reading comprehension exercises that require convergent and divergent thinking.								✔	
Snooper Troops. Consists of a detective game that requires taking notes, drawing maps, classifying and organizing information, and reasoning skills.			✔	✔			✔	✔	

				Process					
	A	M	ORG	O	P	PR	PJ	R	S
Using Context Clues: Levels D and E.								✔	✔
Mindpower II: Thinking Skills in Reading and Language Arts.		✔	✔				✔	✔	
Ant Farm							✔	✔	
Block Construction					✔			✔	
Blockers and Finders I & II			✔				✔	✔	
Interpreting Graphs							✔		
Memory Machine		✔							

Using Context Clues: Levels D and E.
Consists of reading comprehension exercises that require using contextual clues to supply missing words in the passage.

Science Research Associates, Inc.
155 N. Wacker Dr.
Chicago, IL 60606

Mindpower II: Thinking Skills in Reading and Language Arts.
Consists of 36 computer lessons such as completing analogies, distinguishing fact from opinion, predicting what fits in a context, and drawing conclusions; requires ordering, classifying, spatial relations, and deduction and inferences.

Sunburst Communications
39 Washington Ave.
Pleasantville, NY 10570-2898

Ant Farm by Edward E. Annunziata and Thomas Prosen.
Consists of a game that requires the use of problem solving strategies of trial and error and the analysis and examination of assumptions.

Block Construction by Robert Kimball and David Donoghue.
Consists of activities that use logic, inference, visual discrimination, and spatial perception to recreate randomly generated shape puzzles.

Blockers and Finders I & II by Thomas C. O'Brien.
Consists of problems involving complex situations to develop collection and organization of data and higher-order thinking.

Interpreting Graphs by Sharon Dugdale and David Kibbey.
Consists of two programs requiring reading graphic information to solve problems.

Memory Machine by Barbara Wood and David Owen.

	Process								
	A	M	ORG	O	P	PR	PJ	R	S

Consists of activities that provide practice in the use of three memory strategies for retention of pictures, shapes, and descriptive statements.

Pathfinder by Sharon Dugdale and David Kibbey.
Consists of exercises in reading graphs for information and requires the skills of logic and problem solving.

Safari Search by Thomas C. O'Brien.
Consists of 12 search activities that involve problem solving strategies and logical thinking.

Ten Clues by Donna Stanger and Tad Wood.
Consists of activities that require reasoning abilities to decipher a message using individual clues.

The Pond by Marge Kosel and Mike Fish.
Consists of a maze game that requires recognition of patterns, generalization, and logical thinking.

What Shape Is That Color? by Edward and Laurie Pattison-Gordon and Judah L. Schwartz.
Consists of games that require devising a rule, analyzing it, and testing to determine if it fits.

Winker's World of Patterns by Thomas C. O'Brien.
Consists of activities that require making inferences to determine the missing part of a pattern.

Chapter 6

Family Based Treatment: A Systemic Model for Involving Families

Mary A. Andrews and James R. Andrews

Families of individuals with traumatic brain injury can be significant participants at every phase of the rehabilitation-lifelong living process. Most writers who discuss traumatic brain injury rehabilitation acknowledge this; several models of family involvement have been suggested.[1,2,3,4] Whether the professional's role is to provide aggressive rehabilitation treatment or lifelong living services,[5] family members can and should be involved at a level and in a manner that is idiosyncratic to their resources and family lifestyle. Rehabilitation that fails to prepare families to interact and communicate with the "new" member with a traumatic brain injury, or which fails to assist families to resume the launching/independence process begun prior to the injury, is incomplete. The purpose of this chapter is to offer a paradigm for services that supports family participation, to discuss the grief process in terms of appropriate professional responses, and to describe a process and specific techniques for involving families on the rehabilitation team.

THE SYSTEMIC PERSPECTIVE

During the early phase of traumatic brain injury treatment the opinions of surgeons, radiologists, nurses, and other medical personnel are of primary importance. Their combined expertise is essential to the well-being of the patient. This phase is medical in nature. Attitudes and opinions of family members and previous experiences of the patient are likely to be less important than the competent decision making of medical specialists.

During the rehabilitation phase of treatment, however, there are many influences that affect progress. These include the amount and type of stimulation, responses of interactants to the patient, reactions of family members and others who have a close relationship with the patient, and the nature and quality of cognitive-communicative experiences. While the resources of the medical-surgical team may be adequate for physical intervention, the resources of the rehabilitation team may not be sufficient to elicit the greatest improvement in cognitive-communicative behavior. There are many ways that this may become apparent. For example, the voices and sounds of persons closest to the patient may be more stimulating than those of professional rehabilitators; previous experiences with family members may trigger richer memories and thought than would be possible for the speech-language pathologist to elicit; emotional reactions by family members may influence the behavior of the client; communication with friends, family members, and others may stimulate interaction more than communication with members of the rehabilitation team (even though the latter might be more skillful in responding in particular predesignated ways); admonitions and rewards from family and friends may be substantially more powerful than the same responses from professional staff members; and patient cooperation and effort may be greater when interacting with siblings, parents, spouses, and children than with the speech-language pathologist. Under these circumstances, typical of the rehabilitation phase of treatment, the different views and ideas of family members become important in order to elicit the greatest amount of change possible.

The Polyocular View

Family members will be capable of being effective participants in treatment when they feel confident and capable, when they know that their views and ideas are respected, and when their contributions are positively regarded by professionals. The act of listening to different perspectives and understanding that each is correct for the person expressing that particular view and using these perspectives to develop creative treatment plans has been referred to as taking a *polyocular view*.[6] Several perspectives on a problem and ideas for intervention may be expressed by family members. The clinician should value each one (including, of course, the clinician's own), attempt to integrate them, extract the most useful ones, and put them together to form a new whole. The result can be expected to be more useful than the ideas generated by one person or even by a group of rehabilitation experts unfamiliar with the patient's pre-injury interests, personality, attitudes, and family interactions.

Defining the System

One of the first tasks of the clinician who chooses to involve family members is to determine the group to be regarded as the unit of treatment. In traditional one-on-one treatment the unit of treatment is the individual. When the treatment team is expanded to include others who will participate in treatment, however, the group of interactants that will be attended to must be de-

fined by the clinician. For most patients the family provides the most appropriate interactive system with which to work. Family, however, should be broadly interpreted to include a variety of people who may or may not all be legally related to the patient but who are particularly significant in the patient's life. In long-term rehabilitation, the transdisciplinary team as well as the family is likely to be an important part of the patient's significant interactive environment.

The defined interactive system becomes the focus of the clinician's attention. Reactions of these individuals may be observed and discussed. Interactions among the members of the group, as they impact upon problems, can be observed and modified. Family members will learn from the clinician and the clinician will learn from family members. Goals will be mutually determined. The communicative patterns of parents, siblings, and, in some cases, extended family members with the traumatic brain injured patient will be recognized and utilized by the clinician to promote change.

Role of the Clinician

Unlike the clinician who works with the patient alone, the family-focused clinician attends to interactions among persons in the defined system as well as to individual characteristics and responses of the patient. As family members react to the problems of their traumatic brain injured member and as family interactions occur, these sequences of behavior are available for the clinician to reinforce, ignore, discuss, amplify, and/or change. In addition, the clinician may demonstrate particularly effective strategies for stimulation or interaction and reinforce techniques that family members use to facilitate change.

Integration of Counseling Techniques

When families participate in treatment they are apt to show emotions, especially when the injury is as life-changing as a traumatic brain injury. Further, clinicians may have to present information that no family member would want to hear (e.g., the patient is not progressing, the patient must leave the rehabilitation center, etc.). Family members may appear to be angry, hostile, denying the seriousness of the injury, overprotective, or oversolicitous. Participation of families must be elicited and maintained if they are to be part of the solution to the multifaceted problems that accompany traumatic brain injury. This requires the use of counseling techniques by the clinician. To be most effective, counseling techniques are integrated into the daily interactions of treatment rather than being stored up and applied during a particular counseling session. The clinician who has counseling skills is likely to be substantially more effective, even if an individual approach were being used, than the professional who does not. While some may view counseling as an educational or information-giving process, we will discuss a particular group of skills that may be applied in different situations throughout the treatment process.[7,8]

THE GRIEF PROCESS

Speech-language pathologists and other professionals who are involved in the rehabilitation of the person with traumatic brain injury are confronted with issues of grieving throughout the treatment process. Events surrounding the initial trauma, early rehabilitation efforts, and transfer to the family home or rehabilitation setting are likely to engender a myriad of family and patient feelings. These grieving and loss responses will appear, disappear, re-emerge, subside, and appear again throughout the life of the person with traumatic brain injury. An understanding of the grieving process will help the professional respond appropriately to family members, enhancing the effectiveness of family involvement.

A variety of models for understanding the grieving and loss process has been developed by specialists in this issue.[9–13] Paul Spanbock[12] suggests five stages that are experienced by the family members of the head injured individual: (1) shock, (2) elation, (3) reality, (4) crises, and (5) mourning. Following is a review of each stage, the behaviors that are likely to be shown by family members, and recommended appropriate professional responses.

Shock/Impact

Family members experiencing the shock of the unexpected and horrifying news that their loved one has been injured may show numbness, disorientation, disbelief, fear, anger, confusion, helplessness, and physical and emotional pain. The clinician cannot precisely predict how these and other feelings will be expressed, but the overwhelming impact of the events surrounding the crisis is clearly evident. Emergency room and acute care personnel naturally focus their attention on the lifesaving measures that must be taken. Early on, however, family members are informed of medical treatment and included in the decision-making process. While medical intervention is taking place it is essential that the professional remain responsive to the needs of the family. This is not an easy task.

As the shock stage unfolds, the professional should practice the skills of silence, empathic listening, and simple presentation of information. Lectures, detailed explanations, and cheerful banter, intended to alleviate the family's pain, may instead exacerbate their distress as they attempt to deal with the reality of the situation. When expressions of feeling are covertly prohibited by professional staff this may be experienced by family members as a denial of their situation. Attempts to provide detailed explanations, when not requested, will likely fall on numbed ears. Instead, the comforting presence of a calm professional who is willing to allow expressions of feeling and waits for family members to request the additional information that they need will be greatly appreciated. When questions are asked by family members these should be answered honestly and as simply as possible. Information that must be given to the family should be expressed in clear, understandable terms with the knowledge that this same information will need to be repeated in the future. Professional jargon should be avoided. Family members should be assured that periodic discussions with the professional will take place so that, as new concerns begin to emerge, they can be addressed.

Elation/Relief

The shock or impact stage is generally short-lived. When the injured person's life is assured, the family enters a brief stage of elation. Death is no longer a concern and hope for a full recovery is experienced by family members. The injured person may still be in a coma but the family is elated their their loved one will not die and the reality of the current physical status is not important. The professional must continue to show a calm empathic presence and respond to family members' hope, while gently reminding them of the reality of the situation. Following is an example of an appropriately empathic statement: "You are so relieved that John is going to live. This is what you have been hoping and praying for. As we continue to monitor his progress we'll develop a better idea of the extent of his injury and what this means for him and for all of you. We can talk about this later, if you wish." The family's joy should not be taken from them but it is also wise to introduce the idea that the ramifications of the injury are still unknown. Family members can be allowed to celebrate since they will soon discover for themselves that their elation is short-lived. Meanwhile, the professional should be careful not to offer false hope.

Reality

Spanbock[12] suggests that reality is the third stage and that this occurs as family members begin to realize that the injury has resulted in deficits that are likely to be permanent. This stage may occur soon after the injury, when the individual begins to emerge from the coma, or may not take place for several months if the injured person remains in a prolonged comatose state. The professional cannot predict when reality will set in. Indeed, the process may be so gradual that no specific reality point can be identified. In addition, individual family members may protect one another from their personal pain by choosing to appear optimistic long after reality has been experienced. This may be viewed, by family members, as a necessary guise to facilitate the recovery of the person with traumatic brain injury.

The professional will be confronted with the family's anger, depression, anxiety, hope/despair, ambivalence, confusion, and guilt. Anger can be an especially troubling emotion since it may be inappropriately focused on professional personnel. Stern and associates[13] describe the anger shown by family members as the family alternates

between hope and despair related to the condition of their comatose member. The miracle of life has been granted but the ability to relate to their loved one as a living person is denied. Professional staff may be accused of incompetence or a more generalized anger may be focused on the professional staff and/or on the family members themselves. Family members of patients who are no longer comatose also show this anger.

Rehabilitation personnel, who are using every means possible to assure the well-being of the traumatic brain injured person, will need to support one another as they muster up an added measure of patience and understanding when dealing with family members who are expressing anger. Usually, the source of the family's anger is the unacceptable situation. Staff should express their understanding of this as kindly as possible. An example of a statement that may be appropriate when anger is expressed is: "You are deeply hurt and angry that this tragedy has occurred. You're angry with us, yourselves, and John since none of us are able to change what has happened. You want to be certain that everything possible is being done. Let me share with you how I am helping John and then I'd like to get your ideas about what else might be needed here." This kind of statement acknowledges the family's anger at the situation and offers an opportunity for the family to become more involved in treatment, giving them something to do as they adjust to the reality that they now must face.

Sometimes, anger is actually a direct request for more information, social support, or linkage to a psychologist or psychiatrist. The clinician should be sensitive to expressions of emotion that convey a desire for additional assistance from other social service resources.

Guilt may be experienced as family members go over the events surrounding the accident and consider how they might have prevented it. "I should have refused to let him buy a motorcycle," "Why didn't I set a better example about drinking and driving?" and "Was he upset because of our fight?" are examples of dialogues family members have with and among themselves as they attempt to make sense out of the tragedy. In addition, the "new" family member is dramatically different from the preaccident member. Cognitive, behavioral, and emotional changes, whether subtle or dramatic, have created a new person that family members may dislike. How can they not feel guilty about disliking this changed person that they had fervently hoped would not die?

The reality stage also engenders depression related to the future life of their family member and the effect that this will have on the family as a whole. The brief period of hope, experienced during the elation stage, often is replaced by a prolonged sense of hopelessness and despair. Families may show these feelings to the professional by withdrawing, expressing anger, crying, developing physical symptoms, and/or by asking questions that appear to be anger statements in disguise.

During this and all stages, as family members are respectfully encouraged to participate in the treatment planning and implementation process, they become aware of efforts being made on behalf of their loved one and experience for themselves the difficult task of rehabilitation. Firsthand experience takes the place of secondhand criticism and the professional-family team struggles together to implement change strategies. As this is done, the professional should do the following: listen carefully to the family's concerns; understand that their wideranging feelings are related to the unacceptable situation, not to the professional; and begin to develop rehabilitative activities in which the family can participate and that fit the family's idiosyncratic resources and needs. This challenging process offers opportunities for change that may help family members face the reality that they must deal with throughout their loved one's lifetime.

Crisis

According to Spanbock,[12] this stage is not the same as the reaction to a catastrophic stressor-event normally associated with the term "crisis." In this context, crisis is used to describe the ongoing difficulty associated with living with a traumatically brain injured person. Crisis, for example, is experienced when the family is faced with the responsibility of deciding how to care for their family member following inpatient treat-

ment. Continually evolving crises can be related to issues associated with cognitive ability, finances, personal care, sexuality, personality changes, relationships with family members, and the reaction of the larger society to their changed family member. These crises keep appearing, like unexpected storms, and the family must learn how to respond to each of them. If the family has developed problem-solving skills prior to the accident, these will benefit them now. If the family has been chaotic and unable to solve problems in the past, these skills will not now miraculously appear.

The family that has been actively involved in rehabilitation efforts prior to this stage will be better able to cope with the crises that emerge since they will have gradually learned to understand and relate to their family member. The sensitive, competent professional who encouraged their participation on the rehabilitative team will have prepared them to strategize for change as they and the patient access supportive services. During this stage families will show self-doubt, exhaustion, and the continuing grief associated with the loss of the dream.[11] The professional will continue to listen empathically to their concerns, develop treatment plans that encourage their participation, offer advice when it is requested, and be ready to link the family and patient to community resources.

Mourning and Redefining the Relationship

Gradually, family members learn how to relate to their new family member. This new relationship is overlaid with mourning as mothers, fathers, wives, husbands, grandparents, siblings, and/or children begin to fully realize that the "old" person has died. The relationship is redefined in a way that accommodates the new member. Family members' energy for personal interests, unrelated to the injury event, begins to be restored. Crises continue to occur, but, if appropriate support has been established, the redefined family is able to continue its developmental journey albeit forever changed. The professional will experience the joys, hopes, renewed energy, and re-emerging grief of family members as rehabilitation services are provided.

Finally, the professional must understand that the grieving process is not traversed in a linear fashion and then completed, never to emerge again. If full recovery is not achieved, mini-grief processes and re-emergence of varying feelings associated with the different stages of recovery will occur throughout the lifetime of the family. This is a normal and expected pattern for families dealing with unwanted disability.

Grieving Process Variations

The professional must not assume that every family and every individual will move through the grieving process in the same manner. The process, though somewhat predictable, is as idiosyncratic as a thumb print. The goal of the professional is to understand the varying stages so that appropriate responses may be made. For example, efforts to redefine the relationship during the shock stage will fail because the family members are not ready to tackle this accommodation effort. Variations based on the process of recovery, the adaptive resources of the family, and individual differences must be acknowledged. If the patient recovers fully, the family will need the same amount of time that the patient needs to return to their pre-injury lifestyle. Since full recovery is the exception, the professional must remain sensitive to the re-emergence of grief throughout the rehabilitation process.

Grieving and the TBI Recovery Process

The unpredictable and idiosyncratic nature of the recovery of the traumatic brain injured individual has a profound effect on him/her and on family members. Family members waiting at the bedside of their comatose member may linger in the reality stage for months or years as they struggle with the ambivalent nature of their situation. As long as hope remains that their loved one will emerge from the coma, the crisis and redefinition stages may remain on hold. Families whose member does recover from coma will define for themselves the point at which they are able to redefine the relationship with their changed member. This may take months or years but is likely to

occur naturally if the family has been enlisted on the treatment team, has been encouraged to express feelings, and has become an integral part of the change process. The professional, then, must not have a preconceived idea of the amount of time each family will need. Instead, sensitivity to the family's idiosyncratic grieving process must remain while the family's active involvement in treatment is encouraged.

Family Resources

Most professionals are intuitively aware of variations in different family responses to traumatic brain injury. Problem solving abilities, economic resources, family and community support, respite options, personal flexibility, and self-confidence all affect family members as they focus their energy on their loved one's recovery. According to McCubbin and Dahl,[14] four important factors appear to determine which families will be able to adapt to stressful life events: (1) the pile-up of stressful events, (2) the family's strengths and resources, (3) the family's coping skills, and (4) the family's definition of the event. A family is likely to be more vulnerable and experience serious turmoil if: more than one stressful event is occurring (e.g., a grandfather is terminally ill, a sister is about to be married, the family's income has recently decreased, and a young adult son has just been seriously injured while driving under the influence of alcohol); the family has few personal and collective resources (e.g., ineffective communication, inadequate income and/or insurance, no extended family support); coping skills are lacking (e.g., they are unable to identify specific problems and implement solutions); and the family views the stressor event as completely outside of their control (e.g., they believe that there is nothing they can do to help and the situation is completely hopeless). Another family, facing an almost identical situation, may be experiencing only one stressor, have adequate coping skills and resources, and adopt a solution-focused perspective. This family will be better able to deal with the continuing crises that they must face.

Families that are lacking in resources will benefit from involvement because they can be helped to recognize and develop their hidden potential, learn coping skills, and gain personal control as they become actively involved in assisting with treatment. The difficult family will be no less difficult when the traumatic brain injured member returns home if they have not been given an opportunity to change during the inpatient treatment process. Coping skills will not magically appear if no help is offered. If, however, they have been persuaded to join the treatment team and have learned how to use their unique abilities to help relate to their changed family member, new behaviors, however small, can be added to their depleted resources. These changes may generalize to other situations as additional accommodation is required. More fortunate families that have adequate resources will also benefit, as will the clinician, since their expertise becomes part of treatment and enhances the speech-language pathologist's treatment planning options.

Individual Differences

Individual responses of family members may vary as significantly as do the responses of different family groups. Every individual will respond idiosyncratically to the loss experienced and is likely to traverse the grieving stages with different pacing and timing. One family member, for example, may deal with grief by keeping expression of feelings inward and maintaining a strong, passive demeanor. He/she may believe that if pain is expressed other family members will be adversely affected. Another family member may appreciate this outward show of strength or may interpret the behavior to mean that the other person is not upset and then feel unsure about his/her own outward expression of grief. Some people are very open to showing disappointment, sorrow, and anger and grieve in a natural, open manner. Conversely, an individual whose life pattern has been to accept disappointment in a controlled, closed manner will continue to show that same behavior as the new distress is felt. An individual whose style is to openly express feelings will continue to respond overtly. The professional must respect these differences and respond with empathy. Family members, in turn, will become aware of their differ-

ences and be offered opportunity to support one another. The professional must never tell an individual how to grieve. Rather, an understanding of the idiosyncratic nature of the grief process helps the professional respond appropriately to the people who are most severely affected by the ramifications of the traumatic brain injury: the patient and the family.

FAMILY BASED TREATMENT

Family Based Treatment is one approach to including family members as participants in the rehabilitation treatment process. The model evolved from the authors' clinical practice as coclinicians at a university speech and hearing clinic working with clients, families, students, and other professionals interested in creating speech-language change. The process and techniques to be described are drawn from both speech-language pathology and family therapy, but the model is designed specifically for speech-language pathologists. The influence of Jay Haley, a family therapist, will be especially evident to the reader familiar with his problem-solving model.[15] The process includes six steps: (1) convene, (2) share an understanding of the problem, (3) agree on changes and set goals, (4) plan treatment procedures, (5) assess change, and (6) terminate and link. The process is described here to provide the reader with a suggested model to be creatively adapted to fit the unique requirements of varying rehabilitation settings.

Convene

The clinician's first task is to convene family members and any significant others that are part of the patient's interactive system. This first meeting can be arranged in a number of different ways.

In acute care settings, family members tend to be readily available since they often spend a great deal of time at the bedside of their loved one. The clinician should talk to the family member who seems most accessible and arrange a time when everyone can be present. It is often tempting to chat informally with one family member rather than involving as many significant others as possible in an intentional way. While a brief unplanned encounter can be a helpful intervention, it is not adequate for establishing the importance of family participation. Often the burden of care falls on the patient's mother or wife. Therefore, it is essential that fathers, siblings, children, in-laws, and others who can participate in treatment and also support the person who may eventually become the primary caregiver be enlisted early on. This, of course, may require a creative approach to scheduling the family meeting.

In inpatient rehabilitation settings, family participation may be a scheduled part of the patient's rehabilitation program. In addition, family members may be welcomed as they participate in ongoing treatment during hospital visits. Again, however, the professional should underscore the importance of family participation by arranging a meeting at a time when most of the family members can attend. Sometimes a telephone call may be necessary to persuade family members that the professional seriously desires their participation.

Some family members may have felt, in the past, that they were an unwelcome nuisance, even though this was not the professional's intended message. In these cases, the clinician must become a "salesperson," emphasizing the benefits that their participation will bring to the patient's current and future well-being.

The first meeting is critical to the ongoing success of the Family Based Treatment model. In some cases, family members will continue to attend all subsequent meetings. In other cases, family and clinician schedules do not permit full participation at all subsequent meetings. Sometimes one meeting is all that can be realistically arranged and future contact is with different subsystems of the family. Nevertheless, when a respectful alliance is established at the first meeting, the clinician then has access to various family members and can call on them as future needs arise.

An important component in the professional's convening efforts is the use of language. Since family members are not accustomed to believing that their expertise is important or desired, the professional's use of language of participation will encourage family members to rethink this belief and to begin to trust that they can be active participants in the rehabilitative system. The following phrases are examples of the use of language of participation in the convening process: "I know that you can tell me a lot about John, and I need your help as we develop a speech-language rehabilitation plan." "I'd appreciate your ideas as we decide how to help John communicate more effectively." "You know what interested John before his accident. I could really use your input as we plan stimulation activities that might benefit him now." These phrases emphasize the expertise of the family and also convey the clinician's desire to use that knowledge to help their family member. Statements that convey the idea that the professional is the expert and that the family has nothing new to offer are not likely to persuade the family that they should be involved.

Share an Understanding of the Problem

There are different ways of thinking about and understanding the rehabilitative problems resulting from traumatic brain injury. Each professional on the rehabilitative team offers different expertise that is necessary for effective treatment. The speech-language clinician's assessment and evaluation are crucial to the development of effective communicative strategies, whether families are included or not. In an individual-based model, however, the family's perspective may be irrelevant. When families participate in treatment it is essential that the clinician understand their perspectives so that their resources can be effectively linked to rehabilitation efforts.

Once the family is convened it is best to begin the meeting with a few joining remarks.[16] A respectful interest in each family member's uniqueness as well as in each person's strong concerns for the traumatic brain injured family member is essential. Joining is accomplished by acknowledging and promoting the family's strengths, respecting the established roles of family members, and by affirming the self-worth of each individual.[17] Reiterating that family members' willingness to participate is appreciated and explaining, again, why the entire family is needed to help with communication change is helpful. Reminding family members that they are experts in many important areas helps to allay any fears they might have about being criticized or ignored.

The first part of sharing an understanding of the patient's problem focuses on the family's knowledge and expertise. The process by which each member of the family describes how the problem is experienced and understood is itself an intervention. That process usually leads the family to a greater understanding of the cognitive and communicative problems of their family member with traumatic brain injury, their personal reactions to the changes, and interventions that each person has attempted. After listening carefully to the family's perspective, the clinician's view of the problem can be described in a way that is meaningful to the family and solutions that accommodate the family's perspective can be suggested. The specific content of the discussion will, of course, vary with the phase of treatment and the physical and psychological state of the patient.

When the family member is in a coma it might be helpful to discuss the types and content of stimulation that different family members could most effectively offer. For example, such stimulation may include particular expressions that characterized premorbid interactions, music, music mixed with the voice of a family member, music played by a family member, and tastes of different substances characteristic of premorbid likes and dislikes coupled with the voices of particular family members. The clinician, too, is likely to offer stimulation and families can offer important suggestions for the type of stimulation, the content of stimulation, and idiomatic expressions that have particular meaning to the client. When the clinician draws upon the resources of the family, learns their suggestions for stimulation, and discusses with the family a specific plan for implementing their suggestions the resulting stimulation is likely to be more effective than that designed by the clinician alone. Thinking about one's own family at different developmental stages may give the clinician additional insight about family participation.

When the rehabilitative process is more advanced, the content of information obtained from families will be different. Whether the primary problem relates to pragmatics of communication, short-term memory, organizational skills, or other

processes, information offered by the family is no less important. The experiences that family members have shared over the years offer a rich resource to the clinician. By learning about these, utilizing suggestions for treatment made by family members, and learning idiosyncratic premorbid characteristics of the patient the clinician has a substantial opportunity to increase treatment effectiveness. Of equal importance is the clinician's and family's continuing ability to develop communicative strategies that can be used effectively by family members in their daily interaction with the patient.

One other factor relative to learning the family's view bears discussion. Not all family members will view the problem, or even solutions, in the same way. The clinician may find differences of opinion between family members that could possibly affect treatment outcome. Sometimes the clinician will be able to summarize them and find a point of accommodation. In a case, for example, where a young wife believes that speech-language treatment is essential and will help, but the patient's father makes statements that indicate pessimism about rehabilitation, the clinician should clearly state the opposing ideas ("Mr. Olson, you feel terrible that this has happened, but are pretty skeptical about planning a treatment program that will work. Mrs. Olson, you're very hopeful that your husband can be helped by rehabilitation and are eager to get started.") and suggest a point of accommodation ("As you both know, John has been hurt very badly. If, after our evaluation today, it seems to us that John might be able to profit from treatment would you, Mr. Olson, be willing to give it a try, partly to satisfy your son's wife's desire and hopes?"). In this example, an accommodation may be found. The father's attitude continues to be respected, but he is asked to participate in treatment in order to help his daughter-in-law, not because his view is considered as wrong. Had his view not been acknowledged and respected, and had treatment begun, his attitude toward the treatment and his willingness to participate would be quite different than could be expected after this brief intervention to which he is likely to agree.

Questions that are asked during the first portion of the interview should be presented from a neutral position.[18,19] This means that the clinician is nonjudgmental in the approach to each person and does not "side" with any one individual. Questions must not be disguised statements or criticisms but should be exploratory in nature and asked with an intense desire to understand the family's perspective of the problems they now face relative to the communicative disorder. We have found the following questions to be useful:

- "What concerns you most about _____'s communication at this time?"
- "How have you tried to help _____?"
- "Have your efforts been successful and, if so, how?"
- "What have you tried that doesn't seem to work?"
- "What are your hopes for _____'s future?"

When these or similar questions are asked, the professional should take time to listen carefully, explore the details of the information, and continually think about how the family's perspective and resources can be linked to change. Questions about the future help the clinician understand the family members' positions relative to the grieving process and open the door for future discussion about reality issues. The information the family brings to the meeting will often be presented from a framework that is different from the clinician's and it is important to remain empathic and respectful throughout.

The second part of the sharing an understanding stage of the family meeting focuses on the clinician's expertise. An evaluation by the clinician, with family members assisting, is performed in order for the clinician to develop a view of the problem. If the patient is in some stage of coma, for example, the responses to various stimuli offered by both family members and the clinician may be evaluated. The clinician should describe the patient's responses and make sure that the family is also gaining insights. It may be helpful to repeat different forms of stimulation in order to demonstrate to the family examples of the patient's responses. In this way, family members learn the clinician's view slowly and have time to process the information just as the clinician is doing. The process of involving family members in

the evaluation allows the clinician to: (1) reinforce family members for their successes and encourage them to participate in treatment, (2) determine the type of interventions that are likely to be most useful as well as those that are unlikely to be successful, (3) empower families as family members see that they have the ability to elicit a behavioral change in their loved one, and (4) prepare families both to interact/communicate and to intervene in natural interactions in the treatment facility and, later, at home.

If an evaluation has been conducted prior to the first family meeting, this information should be shared with the patient and family, using nontechnical terms and demonstrating the patient's abilities whenever possible. The goal of the first part of the interview is to gather as much data as possible in order to design appropriate interventions that make sense to the clinician and family and that will help the patient.

Agree on Changes and Set Goals

When family members have had an opportunity to express their own views and concerns, offer and try out suggestions for treatment, and learn about the clinician's view of the problem they are in a good position to participate with the clinician in setting goals. Most typically, families will want the clinician to suggest changes that the clinician believes will be most appropriate and to set specific behavioral goals. Even then, however, the clinician should suggest these goals based as much as possible on family concerns and ask the family members whether or not they agree. This simple process of asking the family to "ratify" the treatment plan, and making alterations if they request, confirms that they, indeed, are part of the treatment team.

In some instances, a particular behavior may be especially desirable to change, from the family members' point of view. For example, seeing the loved one eat, acknowledge the family's presence, say a word, and so on, may have special significance. If possible, the desired behavior should be incorporated into the treatment plan. If prerequisite behaviors need to be accomplished first, the sequential plan should be explained to the family members so that they understand that the behavior they want so much is, indeed, a goal that is being approached in a necessarily step-by-step manner.

When family members participate in treatment it is necessary for the clinician's expertise in communication disorders to be linked with the family's resources in order for the family to intervene most effectively. The clinician's internal process of making knowledge usable to a family by planning goals and treatment according to the family's lifestyle, their successful attempts to help their family member, and family roles, rules, and hierarchy is referred to as *creative strategizing.*[8]

It is important for both the patient and the family to experience success. Just as the clinician reinforces patients for behaviors that are desirable, when families participate in treatment the clinician shapes and recognizes their abilities to effect change in their member. The importance of writing goals based upon family strengths and abilities becomes evident when family members are full participants on the treatment team.

Plan Treatment Procedures

In the Family Based Treatment model, families participate in the treatment process through carrying out carefully planned assignments. Assignments are based on both the needs of the client and the particular strengths and abilities of family members. The clinician's role is to develop assignments that fit the resources of the family and the rehabilitative needs of the patient. Assignments can be arranged into three categories and are designed to help family members: (1) notice or pay particular attention to one or more aspect of communication, (2) intervene in a particular way, or (3) monitor progress related to a specific goal. We call these *noticing, intervention,* and *assessment* assignments.

An example of a noticing assignment to family members of a patient in a coma might be: "When you're visiting John, pay particular attention to the stimuli that he responds to most vigorously. Keep a written list of examples so we can talk about them when we get together next Thursday." Other examples are: "Notice what's going on in the room when Roger seems to be monitoring his speech. Pay attention to surrounding noise, the

amount which you and others are talking, his degree of fatigue, and so on. Write down some examples of circumstances that seem to be best for him so we can discuss them next week"; "Bill is beginning to spontaneously say some words. Write down the words you hear him use spontaneously and pay attention to what you do and say to him immediately after he says a word."

An intervention assignment is one in which family members are asked to do something. For example, "When Bill says a word, repeat the word once or twice and reward him by letting him know that you are pleased." Or, "When Keith opens his eyes, move closer to him, look at him, gently touch him, and repeat what you had just done prior to his opening his eyes." Or, "Talk about Joan's sisters and brothers as you show her photos from the family trip you took last summer."

When progress is noticed, especially by family members, an assignment to assess treatment effectiveness may be given. These assignments are similar to noticing assignments, but they have the particular purpose of assessing change and calling change to the attention of family members. These are especially effective when family members indicate that they have noticed progress in the patient. After discussing what the family observed, when they observed it, the circumstances of the situation, and showing genuine pleasure in the new behavior and their attention to it, an appropriate follow-up is to assign the family to pay particular attention to that new behavior and to report back on how often it occurred and how they elicited the behavior. Another use is to determine the effect of a particular intervention. In the case of a traumatic brain injured man with a dysarthria, for example, we assigned his family to "pay attention to whether George's speech is more intelligible when he paces himself by tapping his foot." This had been a previous assignment based upon what appeared to be an effective intervention. We were unsure about whether it was useful outside of the clinic setting, however, and the family's attention to the assignment helped determine its utility.

Assess Change

Subsequent family sessions consist of a review of the assignment and its appropriateness, usefulness, and degree of success. In addition to discussing the assignment, it is especially useful for family members to enact (i.e., carry out) the assignment so the clinician can comment and reinforce those family behaviors that are especially helpful and useful. After the assignment has been enacted under direction of the family, the clinician will likely want to try it also in order to experiment with modifications which may nudge the change process forward.

Frequency of contact between family and clinician will vary with each patient and with the patient's stage of recovery. So too will the formality of the meeting. In the early phases of treatment, frequent contact may be necessary and appropriate. Later, as family members become knowledgeable members of the treatment team and as the situation stabilizes, strategizing sessions may be needed less frequently. The clinician's commitment is to treatment effectiveness and full family involvement rather than to a prescribed number of family meetings.

Termination and Linkage

The decision to terminate treatment, affected by treatment realities, is made in collaboration with the family. At some point in the treatment process the patient will be transferred to another medical facility, to a rehabilitation center, to a long-term care facility, or home to live with the family. These moves to different care settings will end the professional's relationship with the patient unless outpatient services continue with the same professional. Termination of family participation, then, will occur when the patient moves to another setting or when the professional and family believe that management of appropriate care is well-established and regular meetings are no longer needed. At the final session, accomplishments are highlighted and the family members are complimented for their involvement on the team. Inclusion of the speech-language pathologist, who

will be continuing services with the patient at a different facility, will enhance the transition process.

When termination of Family Based Treatment occurs the clinician and family will realize the full benefit of the approach. Family members will understand the rehabilitative needs of their family member. They will be prepared, in part, for the complicated task of accessing and maintaining community services because their ability to assess the benefit of activities that help the rehabilitation process have been enhanced. Unlike the unfortunate families who approach this transition completely unprepared for what lies ahead, they will have learned to develop a problem solving approach to the continuing needs of their family member. The cognitive, emotional, behavioral, and social abilities of the patient as well as the family's resources will, of course, continue to powerfully affect their lives together. They will, however, be empowered to integrate rehabilitative efforts into the natural context of the family environment.

CONCLUSION

Traumatic brain injury powerfully impacts the affected individual as well as the family. The professional who chooses a systemic approach to treatment recognizes the importance of adopting a polyocular perspective, defining the treatment system to include family members, and integrating counseling techniques into the treatment process. When the clinician understands the grieving process and responds appropriately to the client and the family members treatment is enhanced. The Family Based Treatment model offers an opportunity to include family members in the rehabilitation process and, therefore, access resources for speech-language change. These changes will carry over into the patient's natural environment and can facilitate the development of lifelong living services.

REFERENCES

1. DePompei R, Zarski J. Families, head injury, and cognitive-communicative impairments: Issues for family counseling. *Topics in Language Disorders*. 1989;9:78–89.

2. Malkmus D. Community reentry: Cognitive-communicative intervention within a social skill context. *Topics in Language Disorders*. 1989;9:50–66.

3. Rollin WJ. *The Psychology of Communication Disorders in Individuals and their Families*. Englewood Cliffs, NJ: Prentice-Hall; 1987.

4. Rosenthal M, Muir CA. Methods of family intervention. In: Rosenthal M, Griffith ER, Bond MR, Miller JD, eds. *Rehabilitation of the Head Injured Adult*. Philadelphia, Pa: FA Davis Co; 1983:407–419.

5. Jacobs HE, Blatnick M, Sandhorst JV. What is lifelong living, and how does it relate to quality of life? *The Journal of Head Trauma Rehabilitation*. 1990;5:1–8.

6. deShazer S. *Keys to Solution in Brief Therapy*. New York, NY: WW Norton; 1985.

7. Andrews M. Application of family therapy techniques to the treatment of language disorders. *Seminars in Speech and Language*. 1986;7:347–358.

8. Andrews J, Andrews M. *Family Based Treatment in Communicative Disorders: A Systemic Approach*. Sandwich, IL: Janelle Publications; 1990.

9. Fortier L, Wanlass RL. Family crisis following the diagnosis of a handicapped child. *Family Relations*. 1984;33:13–24.

10. Kubler-Ross E. *On Death and Dying*. New York, NY: Macmillan; 1969.

11. Moses K. Dynamic intervention with families. *Hearing-Impaired Children and Youth with Developmental Disabilities: An Interdisciplinary Foundation for Service*. Washington, DC: Gallaudet College Press; 1985.

12. Spanbock P. Understanding head injury from the families' perspective. *Cognitive Rehabilitation*. March/April 1987:12–14.

13. Stern JM, Sazbon DL, Becker E, Costeff H. Severe behavioural disturbance in families of patients with prolonged coma. *Brain Injury*. 1988;2:259–262.

14. McCubbin H, Dahl BB. *Marriage and Family: Individuals and Life Cycles*. New York, NY: John Wiley and Sons; 1985.

15. Haley M. *Problem Solving Therapy*. San Francisco, Ca: Jossey-Bass; 1987.

16. Minuchin S. *Families and Family Therapy*. Cambridge, Mass: Houghton Mifflin; 1974:123–125.

17. Simon FB, Stierlin H, Wynne LC. *The Language of Family Therapy: A Systemic Vocabulary and Sourcebook*. New York, NY: Family Process Press; 1985:203–204.

18. Fleuridas C, Nelson T, Rosenthal D. The evolution of circular questions: training family therapists. *Journal of Marital and Family Therapy*. 1986;12:113–127.

19. Tomm K. Interventive interviewing: Part III. Intending to ask circular, strategic, or reflexive questions. *Family Process*. 1988;27:1–15.

Index